BREAST CANCER BLACK WOMAN

EDWIN T JOHNSON, MD

Van Slyke & Bray
Montgomery, Alabama

About The Cover

The art work on the cover comes from a greeting card, circa 1965 (painter unknown). It depicts a youthful and an older black woman as they sit together, perhaps discussing the commonplace subjects of the day. The women are dressed with color and spark, and yet they remain reserved and demure. The lines of the older woman speak of age and sagacity. The younger woman appears alert and fresh, attentive to the admonitions and guidance of her elder. These are the women who cradle our future. Both are vulnerable to breast cancer. They deserve, nay, command! our respect and protection.

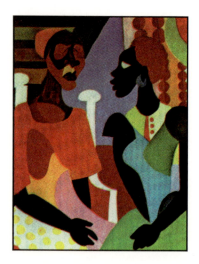

ISBN: 0-9635435-1-2   Library of Congress Catalog No. 98-86265

Manufactured in the United States of America.   First Edition Copyright © 1993

With the unwavering support and editorial skills of my wife, Helen, and the loving encouragement of Niamaat, this book is

Dedicated to the African-American woman, many times found teetering along the fringes of the health care delivery system, and offtimes forced into the role of catch as catch can.

BREAST CANCER
BLACK WOMAN

TABLE OF CONTENTS

FOREWORD ix

PREFACE xi

Preface to the First Edition xiii

INTRODUCTION xv

Introduction to the First Edition xix

CHAPTER ONE 1
WHEN THE SHOE'S ON THE OTHER FOOT

CHAPTER TWO 15
WHERE IT ALL BEGINS

CHAPTER THREE 27
A CASE FOR SHERLOCK HOLMES

CHAPTER FOUR 53
THE FICKLE FINGER OF FATE

CHAPTER FIVE 77
WHEN BREAST CANCER IS ALL IN THE FAMILY

CHAPTER SIX 85
A NEEDLE IN THE HAYSTACK

CHAPTER SEVEN 101
IN THE SHADOW OF TUSKEGEE

CHAPTER EIGHT 107
NO NEWS IS GOOD NEWS, RIGHT? WRONG!

CHAPTER NINE   117
THE BATTLE PLAN

CHAPTER TEN   145
SISTER TO SISTER

CHAPTER ELEVEN   155
HIS EYE IS ON THE SPARROW

CHAPTER TWELVE   177
LIGHTS, CAMERA, ACTION

APPENDIX A   195
NATIONAL BREAST CANCER ADVOCACY ORGANIZATIONS

APPENDIX B   197
AFRICAN-AMERICAN BREAST CANCER SURVIVOR GROUPS

APPENDIX C   199
STATES WITH INFORMED CONSENT LAWS

APPENDIX D   201
SELECTED LIST OF BREAST CANCER CLINICAL TRIALS

REFERENCES   213

INDEX   235

FOREWORD

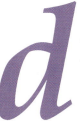

during the year, 1997, an estimated 185,000 new breast cancers were diagnosed. We must continue to stress breast-self examination (BSE), yearly examination by a physician, and increased use of mammography.

In this book, BREAST CANCER/BLACK WOMAN early detection is stressed along with the exchange and dissemination of information to improve survival. This is most important among African-American women who are disproportionately victimized by this disease.

As a community health problem, breast cancer remains a dilemma that demands the best in cooperation among women and their caregivers. There are many aspects of breast cancer that are touched on in this book that will be helpful to women as they work with their physicians to overcome this most common cancer among women.

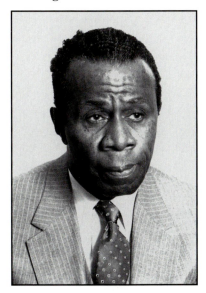

Earl Belle Smith, MD FACS
Distinguished Emeritus Professor of Surgery
Oncology Specialist
University of Pittsburgh College of Medicine

PREFACE

breast cancer is a devastating enemy for American women, especially for black women. In spite of all the knowledge and modern technology available today, African American women continue to suffer the highest mortality compared to the general population, and the highest incidence under forty years of age. Consequently, dissemination of breast cancer information to black women is crucial. This book, BREAST CANCER/BLACK WOMAN is an important step in that direction.

Many of us have been intimately involved with someone who has been touched by this disease. We often discover it in women of childbearing age and, when fatal, this disease deprives not only a family, but a community of irreplaceable benefits.

The cause of black women being disproportionately affected is not known. Genetics, environment, and nutrition have been implicated. But, whatever the cause, we *do* know that if breast cancer is detected early and appropriate measures taken, morbidity and mortality are significantly decreased. One of the major reasons that cancer is not detected early is the lack of information.

Black women must become more diligent in performing self-examinations, obtaining mammograms, and obtaining knowledge about this condition. Many women, particularly those hampered by socioeconomic constraints, are still not having mammograms, doing self-examinations, or getting regular checkups. We must lobby our government and the community to address these needs.

Let us get the message out through our churches, community centers, schools, beauty salons, and all places where black women come together. We can start with BREAST CANCER/BLACK WOMAN. Absorb this information and pass it on.

Remember, what happens to one of us affects all of us. There is a Universal Power through which we live, breathe, and have our purpose. When we acknowledge God (good) and tap into that power, we will be able to love ourselves and thereby love all human kind. The information offered in BREAST CANCER/ BLACK WOMAN represents a segment of that positive force that can lower the destructive effects of breast cancer in all women, especially black women.

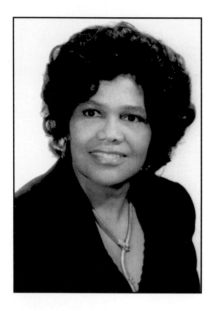

Edith Irby Jones, MD
Past President, National Medical Association

PREFACE TO THE FIRST EDITION

BREAST CANCER IN BLACK WOMEN
condensed from an article by Louis W Sullivan, MD
former Secretary of Health and Human Services

every year more ..women die from breast cancer because they do not receive mammograms and breast exams as often as they should. One out of every nine women will be diagnosed with breast cancer... This year (1992) an estimated 46,000 women will die from breast cancer...1500 more than in 1991, and 180,000 new cases will be discovered.

But breast cancer is particularly devastating in our nation's black women. ....Breast cancer is currently the leading cause of cancer death for African-American women. The National Cancer Institute estimates that over 44,000 black women died from breast and cervical cancer in the last decade.

Only 58 percent of African American women 40 and older have ever received a mammogram. Within the next decade, the lives of more than 13,000 black women could be saved by simply getting regular mammograms and clinical breast examinations.

..when detected early...breast cancer can be treated with radiation or chemotherapy which can reduce the need for radical surgery....90 percent of women who are diagnosed early...will survive breast cancer...

...too many women think it won't happen to them and delay regular clinical breast examinations and mammograms until it is too late.....

Learn and practice monthly self-breast examination...
The cost of breast cancer screenings are between $50 and $150. ...there are ...organizations..and other agencies that have low-cost or free mammography services....

If you have never had a breast exam, don't put it off any longer. Early breast cancer detection can be a choice between life and death. For your sake choose prevention and early detection. Choose life.

BREAST CANCER/BLACK WOMAN was written to help you make the right choice now!

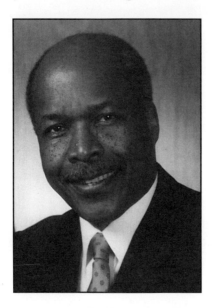

Louis W Sullivan, MD
President, Morehouse School of Medicine
former Secretary of Health and Human Services

INTRODUCTION

During his lifetime, Martin Luther King Junior showed us the Rubicon to the promised land. At every opportunity he preached the power of love and sharingto a people groping for survival. He left examples and sign posts for us to follow. Love was the key, and sharing was the action--to be expressed in deed as well as in word.

Dr King shared his intellect, his counsel, his time, and freely gave his life to humankind. His life represented a selfless expression of love.

If we hope to fulfill the legacy of Dr King, each of us, in our allotted days, must share any talent or information that we possess, that may benefit and uplift the whole. We must do whatever it is in our individual capacity to do, to bring our people closer to the dream. As Dr King said: "Everyone can serve".

With that simple notion, of making life better for the whole, of moving our people closer to the promised land, this second edition of **BREAST CANCER/BLACK WOMAN** was composed.

Since the first edition was printed five years ago, a revolution among black women has begun to unfold. Black women all over this country are taking charge of their lives. They are more in tune with their health and are showing determination to take advantage of the breakthroughs in medical care.

Nevertheless, black women remain more vulnerable than ever to breast cancer. Recent data (1989-1993) reveals that while breast cancer mortality decreased 6% for white women, mortality increased 3% for black women. In 1995 the mortality rate for black women was 16% higher than for white women; and before the age of forty breast cancer mortality for black women is twice that of white women. This gap is caused, in part, by a lack of information, and, to that end, **BREAST CANCER/BLACK WOMAN** has been updated and revised.

The purpose of this second edition is to assist black families in asking questions, and making treatment decisions along with their physicians. To guide the reader in making intelligent choices, four new chapters have been added and others have been modified and updated.

Chapter Five, "When Breast Cancer is All in the Family", is devoted to the genetics of breast cancer. I believe that this is important for black women to understand, since I suspect that a genetic basis for breast cancer is an important component among black women. Only extensive research will tell us for sure; but the signs are there. In the meantime black women should be aware of breast, ovarian, colon, and prostate cancer occurring in their close relatives.

Chapter Seven, "In the Shadow of Tuskegee", covers the importance of clinical trials in the pursuit of new methods of treatment. Black women have been under-represented and often ignored. The importance of primary health care providers in restoring faith in black women to participate is emphasized. A full discussion of what goes into a clinical trial and the various phases involved is outlined.

Black women must have insight in all of the ramifications of clinical trials and then decide based on their personal preferences whether or not to participate.

Chapter Ten, "Sister to Sister", is a

salute to breast cancer survivor groups. Black women have organized to provide mutual support and the exchange of information. Indeed, there is evidence that depression can be controlled and thwarted when women interact in this way.

Chapter Eleven, "His Eye is on the Sparrow" is a collection of selected conversations with breast cancer survivors who have opened their hearts to discuss their fears and pain, their coping strategies, and their joy of victory.

Chapter Three "A Case for Sherlock Holmes" has been expanded to explain in more detail how the diagnosis may be made with the needle biopsy which is rapidly replacing the open biopsy as a preferable alternative. Other promising diagnostic methods, especially for younger women with dense breasts, are also examined.

Chapter Four "The Fickle Finger of Fate" is a discussion of breast cancer risk factors. I explain at some length proliferative breast disease as a risk factor, since this entity is not uncommon in black women. The fact that induced abortion appears to be related to breast cancer more so in black women is also disclosed.

Chapter Nine "The Battle Plan" concerning treatment options has been revised to inform the reader regarding current therapies, and how one can decide on the best personal treatment alternative.

BREAST CANCER/BLACK WOMAN is for every breast cancer survivor, every black woman who has had a family member with breast cancer, and every black woman who has known a friend or acquaintance with breast cancer. For every woman, information is the first step to survival. Decisions regarding breast cancer must be based on knowledge, rooted in information. I invite you to read and share **BREAST CANCER/BLACK WOMAN**—to expand your personal knowledge with information that will heighten your vigilance, and augment your survival tactics. In the final analysis, this book is simply another sign post, that must be observed and shared as together we seek the path to the promised land.

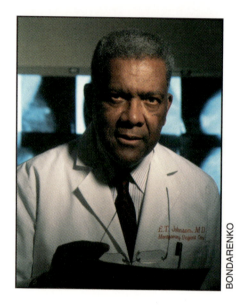

Edwin T Johnson, MD
July 1999

INTRODUCTION TO THE FIRST EDITION

Several years ago I had the occasion to participate in a *Health Education Fair* sponsored by one of those missionary circles that are found in every black Baptist church. I could have chosen to speak on hypertension or sickle-cell anemia, both important topics in the black community. But I had recently operated on a twenty-six year old black woman with breast cancer, and I decided this was an opportunity to remind these church members of the danger signals of breast cancer and the importance of early detection.

As I began to review the literature in preparation for my talk, I was surprised to learn that black women, young and old, were contracting breast cancer at an ever alarming rate, especially in the 30 to 50 year old age group. At the same time I found that the incidence was stabilizing among whites.

I also discovered that more black women with breast cancer had a spreading malignancy when first discovered; and fewer white women had advanced breast cancer when first seen. So the cure rate for black women was lower. Even when breast cancer was detected at a comparable stage, the chance for survival, for obscure reasons, was much worse among black women. And finally, I found that black women were caught up in myth and mis-information regarding cancer in general and breast cancer in particular.

Obviously, I had to conclude: Black women are at special risk.

Instead of just a general review of the danger signals of breast cancer, I felt this

'Health Education Fair' was a perfect opportunity to give these black women information that pertained to them directly. As far as I could observe there was little concerted effort on the global scene to warn the black community of their peculiar vulnerability to breast cancer.

Certainly current resources available to the community were inadequate to address many of the common health issues facing black people, much less focus on breast cancer. But individual effort might make a difference. If speaking to small groups such as this health fair had merit, then addressing a wider audience should have an even greater impact. Perhaps a book directed towards black women and their families was part of the solution.

I reviewed the medical literature, and sought the opinion of leading authorities of the day. I talked to nurses and therapists. I interviewed cancer patients and their families; and pondered my own personal surgical experience in treating breast cancer, which was occasionally rewarding, but too often too late and tragic.

The idea of a book? Why not! A book that would alert black women and not frighten them, would counsel and not preach. A book that would inform and challenge. A book with a title that was not fancy but would get right to the matter. Aha! But how to go from an idea into reality—from blank sheet to something tangible?

There were no short cuts. It was a process of distilling the information, rewriting, reworking, rethinking, rechecking, updating, and repeating the process again and again.

Eventually my thoughts were shaped and crystallized into this volume: **BREAST**

CANCER/BLACK WOMAN. In the first chapter it was necessary to fictionalize patient names and events to satisfy editorial constraints. Chapter One is a fictional discussion which was based on numerous actual interviews with real breast cancer patients.

The goals of **BREAST CANCER/BLACK WOMAN** are threefold:

The **first** goal is to cut through the maze of misinformation and make the reader aware that breast cancer can be cured when discovered early.

The **second** goal is to emphasize that every woman should play a vital integral part in detecting breast cancer at an early favorable stage.

The **third** goal is to encourage black women to evaluate the options now available in the care of breast cancer and participate in treatment decisions.

The African American Woman is at special risk for Breast Cancer. To increase her chance for cure and survival she must have the right information. Here is that information.

Edwin T Johnson, MD
December 1993

CHAPTER ONE

WHEN THE SHOE'S ON THE OTHER FOOT   The Patient's Point of View

physicians and care givers must continually ask themselves the question, 'How would I respond if I were the patient? How would I want to be treated? What if the shoe was on the other foot?'

That question has been constantly before me as a physician whenever I've been called upon to give an injection, or pass a tube, or repair a laceration or in some way to inflict discomfort.

When a particular procedure promises to be uncomfortable or downright painful, I tell the patient, "I'm pretending I'm doing this to myself, so you know I'll be careful."

It's amazing how one can reduce the discomfort with that simple thought. It might mean waiting a few minutes to locate a smaller catheter, or using a smaller needle, or taking the time to numb the throat when passing a stomach tube. All sorts of things come to mind when you consciously put yourself in the patient's shoes.

Have you ever noticed how bad it hurts when someone uses a pin to remove a splinter from your finger? But when you do it to yourself, it doesn't hurt nearly as much. That's because you automatically do whatever you can to avoid pain that you will feel while you remove the splinter from your own finger. It's simply human nature.

I believe all caregivers should respond in human terms to that question, 'What if I were the patient and the shoe was on the other foot.' For surely as we live, the toll of time will eventually place all of us in that circumstance.

This chapter is for the care-givers—not only the medical professionals, but even more for the patients' loved ones—the husband and off-springs, the well-wishers, the friends, even the casual acquaintances. It's time for all of us to be caring givers, to appreciate the breast cancer dilemma through the experience of the patient. Hopefully this awareness will heighten our empathy and sensitivity and help us lend our support and understanding in finding a coping strategy.

Before 1975, treatment options for breast cancer were not generally explained to the patient by most surgeons; and, in those days that was perfectly permissible. When a patient was anesthetized, she understood that if the biopsy was positive for cancer, radical surgery was to be done before waking her. If the patient awoke without a breast, obviously there was cancer. And that was acceptable treatment. Few doctors asked the question, 'How would I want to be treated?'

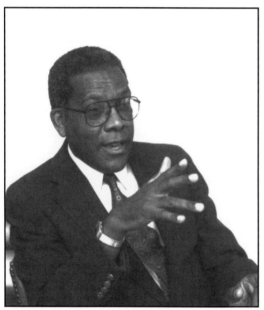

The doctor...is required to make breast cancer patients aware of...treatment options. Women must be involved in making treatment choices.

Nowadays, however, in several states the doctor, by law, is required to make breast cancer patients aware of all available treatment options.[3] See Appendix C. Medical information is now available to the public as never before. People are generally more informed, and often insist on making their own decisions, or at least be a part of the decision making process. The doctor today, to be in step with the times, must give his patient that option. A new era of doctor-patient relationship is upon us. Patients no longer need to accept whatever is offered, oblivious of other choices. It is no longer acceptable to let questions go unanswered or simply to 'observe' a breast lump because the doctor said so. The most common medico-legal allegation filed against physicians is due to the failure to diagnose breast cancer.[2]

Women must be alert and doctors must be aggressive in uncovering breast cancer. This is particularly true in the case of black women under age 35 where breast cancer occurs one and a half times as often as in the white population.[1] Obviously black women and all women must be informed regarding available treatments and involved in the making of sometimes difficult choices.

Hopefully information in this book will provide women and their families with a better understanding of breast cancer, particularly in the black community, and encourage them to openly discuss their needs and concerns with their health providers and to be an active participant in treatment decisions.

I interviewed a number of black women who had been treated for breast cancer before 1975. None of them was my personal patient. I found them through oncology nurses, social workers, medical colleagues and simply word of mouth. I learned of their experiences with their doctors, the hospital staff, the reaction of their husbands and family, and their adjustment in the work place. I believed that the viewpoints of black women from different age groups and backgrounds who had actually lived through those trying days should be recorded and passed on to enhance our sensitivity and make all of us more understanding and aware of this cancer epidemic.

I reviewed my notes from numerous interviews and discovered that none of these women were given any real opportunity to participate in their treatment decisions; and several had stories of depression and misgiving. Others related insensitivity at the hands of medical professionals and lack of support from loved ones.

I decided to incorporate these viewpoints into three fictional women of diverse backgrounds and age groups, and allow them to openly describe their impressions, and talk about how they coped with their cancer—to convey the psychological impact of breast cancer.

Peggy Thornton was a 37-year-old single parent who had discovered breast cancer some time in 1968, had a mastectomy in 1970, and then faced an emotional roller coaster of fear, disgust, divorce and finally accommodation. She survived an ordeal and now, for several years has worked as a bank officer.

Mrs Foster, on the other hand, was in her late sixties, overweight, bent with arthritis, and on medication for high blood pressure. She'd been married for over 40 years and had raised a family before finding a knot in her breast and undergoing mastectomy about 1972.

Mrs Beatrice Robinson, a 52-year-old housewife who had had a mastectomy in 1974 had adjusted fairly well and had good support from family and friends. She blamed her doctor for not finding her cancer.

Let's pretend these fictional characters, some time in 1975, gathered in my office at my invitation to talk about their experiences. Here are some excerpts from that discussion based on notes from actual patients:

"In a few days I'm scheduled to speak on breast cancer and the black family. I would like to relay some of the problems faced by patients with their doctors and with the hospital staff. Tell me about attitudes you faced at home and on the job. I want you to help me to understand what it's like when the shoe's on the other foot."

Peggy Thornton spoke up right away. "Well, I think it's high time somebody tried to find out what patients feel and how we do after the surgery is all over. I'll be happy to tell you how I got along. I had this white doctor. They're supposed to be so good, no offense, Dr Johnson; but that doctor didn't tell me a thing. He was just too cold and impersonal. I didn't even know he was going to remove my breast."

It would seem that Mrs Thornton was not pleased with her doctor. And this is the dilemma I've heard time and time again. Black women and their families naturally want the best medical care possible; and black folks, in general, actually believe the white man's ice is colder. We may be able to out-run, out-jump, out-sing and out-dance the white man, but when it comes to serious business, so many of us make haste to submit our treasure and our bodies to the man, having been taught in so many subtle ways that the white pilot, the white lawyer, or anything white has more innate knowledge or skill. In the same vein, many black women opt for a surgeon who looks like Jesus and quickly overlook his cool detached attitude. I recall patients who have sought a second opinion (code for preferring a white doctor), only to be put to sleep and then actually operated on by a doctor in training, while her surgeon looked over the trainee's shoulder or retreated to the lounge for a Coke or cigarette.

I also remember vividly being called as a friend of the family to give my opinion regarding a desperately ill patient with liver cancer at the VA Hospital in San Francisco. The patient had obviously expired. I examined my friend carefully. He was still hooked up to IV fluids and a mechanical breathing apparatus. The nurses had been waiting about 30 minutes for a doctor to come and pronounce the patient dead, and in the interim the family had called me at my office to come and, I thought, to give my opinion. I left an office full of patients to be at the side of this family in this crisis; and I tried to explain as tenderly as possible that this good husband and father was gone. No one said a word. There was no emotion. The drip of the IV continued. The grind of the respirator and the rhythmic heave of the thorax proceeded. I suspected the wife was in shock, so I whispered again to the patient's brother, "I believe he's gone, Robert."

"We're waiting for the doctor," replied Robert.

After another 15 minutes or so, watching the chest go up and down, Dr Jesus breezed in followed by two nurses holding medical charts. He took one look, waved his stethoscope across the chest, and exclaimed to the group, "This man is dead." He looked at the nurses, "Remove the respirator and IV's." And then he was gone, no personal words to the family. Nothing.

In an instant the seven or eight family members around the bed let up a holler. You talk about wailing and gnashing of teeth. They hugged each other, screamed and sobbed. In the melee someone thanked me for coming. And I slipped away feeling my ice was not quite as cold as I thought it was.

Therefore I understood very well where Peggy was coming from. Black physicians immersed in the quagmire of medical racism on a daily basis, must also tolerate a cool aloofness from white colleagues. But this was not a time to voice my own opinion or experiences. This discussion was about learning from these women — how they coped and responded to their own personal experiences. So I proceeded.

"Alright ladies let's begin by throwing out a question for you. How did you happen to discover the lump in your breast. Was it your own finding or did a doctor or nurse find it on routine examination."

Mrs Robinson, who had a mastectomy in 1974, began to speak. "I'd been going to my doctor for diabetes but he never checked my breast. I had to find it myself. I was just lying on the couch watching television. I guess I was scratching or rubbing my breast when I felt this knot."

Again, I sensed that the doctor or the system was being blamed. "How long had you been going to that doctor for diabetes, Mrs Robinson?"

"Oh, for years."

"And he never gave you a complete examination?"

"He probably did a long time ago, but nothing regularly. He would just check my sugar and write prescriptions."

"Tell us about this knot you found."

"I didn't think too much of it at the time. But I noticed it a few days later while in the bathtub. I told my husband and he thought I should have it checked. I knew it couldn't be a cancer because it didn't hurt or nothing. Then I kind of forgot all about it until I noticed it was growing."

"And how long did that take."

"I guess it was about six months later."

"Did you tell your doctor then?"

"No I didn't. I kind of thought it might be an infection or something. I guess I was hoping it wasn't a cancer. I was hoping it would go away. But then my arm started swelling and I finally told my doctor. He referred me for surgery right away."

"How much time passed between the time you first noticed the lump and finally had surgery."

"It must have been over a year, Doctor Johnson."

"But you saw your doctor for diabetes and probably other things during that time!"

"Yes, but be didn't check my breasts and I guess I didn't tell him about it. Don't ask me why. I know I should have," she smiled.

I suppose it's easier to blame the system, I thought. But shouldn't the patient take some responsibility also?

"You had the breast removed, I understand. Were you given any other treatment choices?"

"No, the surgeon said that this was the best way to go and I thought that he, being the doctor, knew best. I never even thought to question anything."

"What about you, Peggy? What were the circumstances when you first noticed something was wrong?"

Peggy Thornton had gone on to complete her degree in business administration since her mastectomy in 1970. She was now in the management training program at one of the leading banks. She was a divorcee and was raising a teenage daughter with the help of her mother, who lived with her.

"I first was aware that a lump was in my breast when I accidentally bumped myself on a sack of groceries I was holding and leaning on, trying to get my key in the front door. It hurt a little and at first I thought I bruised my breast, but later I checked and found this knot. It didn't feel like a bruise and I immediately thought of cancer. But would you believe I was too scared to see a doctor or even to talk about it. When I did go to this black doctor, his receptionist asked me right out in front of everyone in the waiting room what my problem was. She was behind a counter but still everybody in the room could hear. I told her I wanted to speak to the doctor privately and she tells me that I had to tell her first. You know how we are when we get a little job. I could have kicked her behind right there, but I was cool. I told her I'd return later but I was so embarrassed I never went back.

"For about a year I kept putting it off and hoping the lump would go away. It didn't seem to be getting any bigger and I guess I really hoped it would eventually go away. Then I got this lump under my armpit, and that's when I mentioned it to my husband."

"How did he respond?"

"Horrible. He was in the middle of working on his Masters degree and trying to hold down a job. Our daughter was only ten and I guess the pressure was too much for him. He just balled me out for not telling him sooner. He just couldn't or wouldn't understand how scared I was even though I knew it was probably a cancer. We weren't getting along too good anyway but we started having more fights. He didn't want to even get close to me. Then my sister told me about this white doctor at the medical center. He was supposed to be a good surgeon and all that. But, Lord knows, he was so cold—I mean chilly!—if you know what I mean (I did). I don't think he ever looked me in the eye once. He said he'd do a biopsy and remove the breast if it was a cancer; but he wasn't sure it was a cancer and not to worry about it. So I didn't really think they were going to cut off my breast even though I signed a consent form. To me that consent form meant: 'I trust you to do the right thing'.

"After surgery I woke up with this huge bandage on my chest. I wasn't hurting much at first, but I was scared. I was so depressed and angry, but what could I do? My husband was acting like a robot. We hardly even spoke when he came to the hospital. I was a mess. My chest looked so bad when they changed the dressing I cried. It was terrible. I had no idea it would look so bad, and the doctor talking about how good it was healing. A radical mastectomy. Can you imagine?

"My little girl wanted to know what was happening. My husband was withdrawn, and my momma talkin' about 'give it time'. My arm started swelling and my shoulder got stiff. The surgeon seemed too busy to give me much time. Even the interns, you know, the student doctors seemed too busy to talk much.

"When I finally got home I couldn't find the right kind of bra for weeks. Clothes wouldn't fit right. I got my hair done, but it didn't look right."

Her eyes rolled up and a sigh whistled through her teeth. "I tell you, for a while it was pure hell."

"Well, we can be thankful you've managed to come this far, Peggy. You've been fortunate to have no residual arm swelling or shoulder stiffness. I think you've shown you've got what it takes to overcome. Now, what about you, Mrs Foster? We haven't heard from you. Tell us how you discovered you had a breast cancer. Did you get the support you thought you needed at home?"

Mrs Foster, plump and gray in a flowered house dress, was almost seventy years old. She seemed content and adjusted in spite of the chronic swelling of her right arm, held in check by an elastic sleeve. She gave us a broad smile.

"You see, Doctor Johnson, I been married about 45 years and me and Jim, my husband, we'd seen a lots together, children all grown and everything. My husband had that prostrate surgery a few years before my surgery, so he couldn't do much in the way of sex anyways, so our relationship didn't really change that much."

I hadn't asked about sex relations, but this simply pointed out that regardless of age, sex is not far from the topic of conversation even at age sixty-nine.

"In fact he was real nice to me when I was sick," said Mrs Foster. "I guess I wasn't looking for him to be mean or nothing. Truth is he's always been good to me. And my children still come around reg'lar—makes it nice. Even when they brings theys children for me to mind."

She smiled broadly again and the rest of us responded.

"Tell us how you found out there was something wrong with your breast?"

"I was dressing—putting on my clothes, when I felt this hard knot in my breast. 'Bout the size of the end of my finger. It didn't hurt or nothin'. (Too many women are falsely reassured because it doesn't hurt). I thought about cancer, but it didn't hurt, so I didn't rush to see about it right away. But I did mention it on my next appointment with the doctor."

"And when was that, Mrs Foster?"

"I saw Dr Carter about a month or so later. I still didn't worry about it being a cancer. He checked me and then he got all excited and started fussing about women carrying around these cancers for years before telling anybody. But he never told me I should be checking myself. How was I to know?"

"I understand. But now you can pass the word to your friends about the importance of checking themselves regularly."

"Tha's right and I do just that. I had my surgery in, I think, 1972, and I'm doing fine. I have a little swelling in my arm but it don't bother me too bad. I can still do all my work and we still go fishin' just about every weekend."

"That's wonderful. You've done very well, Mrs Foster. Now here's another question for somebody. Did any of your doctors sit down and explain other choices of treatment? Mrs Robinson—Peggy?"

"Well, no. My doctor just said what had to be done and I went along with it. I figured he would know best," said Mrs Robinson.

"I already told you I didn't even know my breast was going to be removed for sure, much less any other possible choices," said Peggy.

"Okay. Peggy, you and Mrs Foster have told us about your husbands' reactions to your surgery. What about you, Mrs Robinson? How did your husband respond?"

"My husband was left in the dark, more or less. He always felt the surgeon avoided talking to him or felt awkward about keeping him informed. Maybe it was because he was a white doctor. We were never told about reconstructive surgery and the doctor never said too much about practical things such as using padded bras or suggest the best way to dress. I think he left it up to the people in rehabilitation and the American Cancer Society ladies that visit after surgery to fill me in on those things. But I learned a lot. At least I know how to pronounce 'prosthesis', now.

"Anyway, we were referred back to my personal doctor, but my husband and I both wished the surgeon himself had gone over all these things and gave us more attention and advice. After all, he wasn't too busy to cut off my breast."

In the 1970-75 period physicians shouldered most of the responsibility of informing and guiding the patient to ancillary services. Today, the doctor depends on agencies and health workers, and delegates many tasks. But the doctor must be sure the patient understands this new team approach.

Mrs Robinson continued, "After my operation, we weren't able to sit down and talk more than five minutes with the surgeon. He never seemed to have time. I made a list of things to ask because he rushed me. At least I thought he did. Even with a list I couldn't get my questions answered. My family doctor told me to call the surgeon if I had any problems. So there you are. I just wish doctors would take a little more time with their patients."

Some things for some patients cannot be delegated. The doctor must understand that too.

"Well, let me voice my view on this. Only a few years ago most physicians, including myself, felt a strong responsibility in making the decisions on a particular line of treatment. After all, the

> Over the past twenty years things have changed dramatically. Today, in 1998, there is more information available to the public than ever before, and patients can learn about various diagnostic methods and treatment options. Certainly every patient has the right to ask questions and participate in therapy decisions.
>
> Now, we have what they call peer review, where doctors monitor the work of their fellow doctors; and there's quality assurance, where doctors and ordinary citizens monitor the activities of doctors. These committees are set up to assure better care and communication between doctor and patient.
>
> Doctors must keep up with new innovations and treatments through continuing medical education and in some cases re-certification. These are all forces that have affected the doctor-patient relationship and the physician must respond to these new constraints and keep the patient and family fully informed or find himself isolated in a precarious position.

When the Shoe's on the Other Foot

patient had no means of judging what was the best treatment; and we believed the patient depended on our guidance. So you must take that into consideration when you tell me that your doctors left you in the dark. Perhaps, if he had spelled out all the options and all the types of procedures and treatments and all the possible complications you would have to be so confused you'd still be in the dark."

"I still think the doctor should explain more," said Peggy. "Doctor Johnson, patients just want to know what's happening. That's all."

"Actually you are right. Most things can be explained in terms that anyone can understand. Certainly we have an obligation to explain to our patients and their families. If the shoe were on the other foot I'm sure we would want the same.

"Now let's see what's next. Oh yes. Did any of you have a visit from someone from the American Cancer Society?"

"Let me tell you about the women from the American Cancer Society, Doctor."

"Yes, the Reach to Recovery Program. Did they visit you Peggy? Was it worthwhile?"

"In a way, I believe it was. I was feeling so bad I needed a shoulder to cry on or at least someone to talk to. Like I said, my husband was out to lunch and my doctor was out in space. But the Reach to Recovery program helped. The person from the American Cancer Society was very nice. She told me about where to get a bra and who to call to compare different styles. She

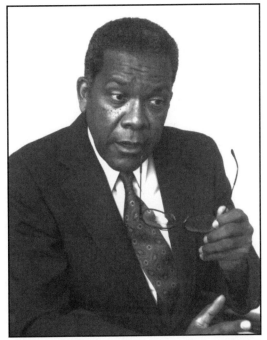

We have an obligation to explain to our patients and their families. If the shoe was on the other foot I am sure we would want the same.

gave me a little pillow to wear in my bra when I was discharged from the hospital. You'd be surprised to know how important it is to have some kind of padding in your bra just to get home from the hospital."

"Did you get a visitor from the American Cancer Society, Mrs Foster?"

"My lady came by and we had a good visit too. She was real polite and told me she was from the American Cancer Society and had the same operation and was doing fine; and she left me some little folders to read."

"Was she a black woman, Mrs Foster?"

"Yes. I think she was about my age too. We talked about families and grandchildren and such. She showed me pictures. And you know, we knew some of the same people. In fact I'd been to her church to a musical program. I talked with her several times after I got home."

Mrs Robinson chimed in, "Those ladies from the American Cancer Society were nice to me too, Doctor Johnson, but some of those nurses and aides I had in the hospital were horrible."

"Tell us about that, Mrs Robinson?"

"Do you know, they let me lay there and I could hear 'em laughing and talking down at their station. Wouldn't answer my buzzer for nothing, and when they did, they'd just leave me for hours before I got a pain shot. And I thought some of them were just too rough when changing my dressing or getting me to walk. Of course they say they have to be rough to get patients to do for themselves. But that's not true, because some other nurses were just as sweet and got me to exercise and walk just as much. I believe some nurses are just cruel and need to suffer themselves before they're allowed to wait on patients. This goes for white and black nurses."

"Of course when we're sick we may be more sensitive and perhaps more demanding, but still there may be some truth in what you say. I know I'm a lot more understanding of a patient with a back sprain, since I sprained by own back.

"I've always felt that black patients expect more out of black nurses, because they identify with them—black and female. They look for those nurturing characteristics found in grandmothers and mothers who cared for them through childhood illnesses. I've been hospitalized more than once myself. Believe me even a *half-mean* nurse (black, white, Asian, or whatever) is a total disaster for a patient in pain.

"Okay now. Someone tell me about how you made out around the house. How'd you cope with going back to work? Let's see now. Mrs Foster, you had your mastectomy in 1972. Tell us about your rehabilitation.

When the Shoe's on the Other Foot

Did you have any complications?"

"Well not too much. My arm and hand stayed real swoll' for a few weeks, my shoulder was stiff and o' course my chest hurt for a long time; but I kept workin' it and wearing that elastic sleeve and eventually everything got better. But I still use an elastic sleeve to keep down the swelling."

"What about follow-up visits to your doctor?"

"Well I saw my doctor every month for a long time."

"Did he seem attentive and understanding?"

"Yes, he did. He wasn't the one that operated. He was just my family doctor, but he watched over me pretty good I think. I'm supposed to go back every six months to get a check on my other breast and get an x-ray."

"Do you recall anything about the hospital and nursing staff?"

"Yes. They all seemed real good. I didn't have no trouble."

"What about going back to work or just resuming your daily activities? Did anyone have trouble coping with that? How did you all get along?"

"That part was just fine," said Mrs Robinson. "My family was real supportive. My husband and I talked a little about plastic surgery, but the mastectomy hasn't seemed to interfere with our sexual relations and I had no problem with my clothes fitting okay, since I used the prosthesis in my bra. We decided not to have any more surgery. I didn't work outside the home, so I didn't have to worry about going out every day to a job."

"And you Peggy. You were working. How did things go when you returned to work?"

"At the time I was working in an insurance office as a clerk. A great big room with umpteen desks and women wall to wall, typewriters, and phones buzzing for eight hours straight. I just felt awkward. Like everybody was looking at me, even though there were partitions between us. My doctor told me that plastic surgery couldn't be done in my case, and I was always aware that so much of my chest was gone—not just my breast, but muscles too. I just felt like people were looking through my clothes.

"It was a pretty good job, but I just up and quit. Everybody just acted differently after my surgery. Somebody would ask me every day how I felt. You know how folks are when they're trying to be nice?"

"Everybody was just too polite all the time. Or else someone wanted to let me know that they knew someone who had breast cancer and how brave they were until the end."

"They did me that way too chile," said Mrs Foster. "Look like I couldn't go to church without some well meanin' soul asking me if I was doin' okay. And do you know people be telling me I looked tired. I declare people don't know what to say. Now that bothered me more'n anything. If the shoe was on the other foot, I believe it'd be a different story."

"Amen to that."

C H A P T E R T W O

VHERE IT ALL BEGINS
Breast Development, Construction and Function

t was HEALTH AWARENESS DAY at a predominantly black inner city community center. The event had been well publicized and the sponsors were happy with the turnout. The Public Health Department, Commission on Aging and several other agencies were represented with booths and brochures. Purveyors of medical information had descended en masse to deliver the message of caution and emphasize the virtue of personal health. Young people were being inundated with the dangers of drug abuse and sexually transmitted diseases. Older folks were getting their blood pressure checked, and lining up for cholesterol testing. It was all about making good choices, and respecting the mind and body. There were posters about diabetes, nutrition, and sickle-cell anemia.

The organizers also planned to cover topics on cancer, especially lung cancer and breast cancer. Lung cancer was a preventable disease, so the dangers of cigarette smoking would be highlighted with videos and talk sessions and handouts.

I was invited to say a few words on breast cancer, since that was an area of special interest to me; and the local chapter of the American Cancer Society was helpful in providing a film on breast cancer that emphasized early detection. I had decided to give a brief talk on the anatomy and function of the breast before showing the film. I was ushered to a small auditorium seating about 150 people. From the rostrum I had a chance to glance over the audience. There were mostly women of all ages. Some were holding small children. Towards the rear of the room I spied a large group of boys and girls—teenagers, laughing and noisy and just being teenagers. A sea of precocious youth, bursting at the seams with energy and life.

Then I was being introduced. "We are happy to welcome Dr Johnson to this segment of HEALTH AWARENESS DAY. He's going to speak on..."

While the introduction continued I had a chance to look at my notes and I took a moment to study the faces before me—a few dull and distracted; but most seemed interested or at least curious. The youth in the rear seemed more interested in each other with subdued chatter and occasional gum popping. Only a few seemed to be interested in what I had to say. Surely, I thought, some would be curious enough to listen in spite of the distractions around them. Who knows? One of these youngsters amid the confusion may one day discover some universal truth that would someday save us all.

"....So let's give Dr Johnson your attention." I stepped to the lectern and began to speak.

"As part of HEALTH AWARENESS DAY, we've been invited to discuss various health issues with you. You've been learning about sexually transmitted disease, sickle-cell anemia and other health issues. Well, in this segment the topic is breast cancer, one of the major cancers—-affecting one in eight women in this country.

"My presentation, the movie, and handouts, will all be stressing the same thing—your responsibility to protect your health and the health of your family. So it's important that you know something about breast cancer, by far the number one cancer in American women.

"The good news is that over 85 percent of breast cancers can be cured if found early. The bad news is that relatively more black women are likely to die of breast cancer. Does anyone have any idea why that is so?"

No one responded. Faces were blank. But the question at least quieted the room and even the teenagers in the back were glancing my way. I continued.

"Too many black women are lost to breast cancer because so many are unaware of the danger signals and too few are being checked on a regular basis.

"Now before we view the film from the American Cancer Society about the danger signals and early detection, let me review some basics.

Let's go back to where it all begins. Let's examine the normal anatomy and function of the breast.

"First, we'll look at the breast through the microscope, so to speak, and examine the various tissues that make up the human breast, such as the glandular structure, the lymph channels, the blood vessels and the underlying muscles. Then we shall review how body hormones affect the normal breast and, perhaps, stimulate cancerous growth. Now relax. I'm not going to try to impress you with high sounding medical words. We'll keep things simple and understandable. And please feel free to ask questions as we go along.

"By way of introduction I shall make a few remarks about the breast development in various animals, and then outline the growth and development of the breast in humans. I have plenty of copies of the presentation for you to take for further study."

Mammals and Breast Tissue

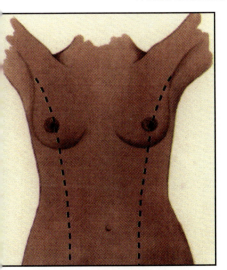

Fig. 2-1. The Milk Ridges. The broken lines represent the position of the milk ridges that are very prominent in the embryo. A nipple and breast tissue may form anywhere along these ridges.

Warm blooded animals that have specialized glands that produce milk are called mammals and those milk-producing glands are called mammary glands. Before birth a continuous thickened ridge develops in the skin along the right and left sides of the embryo's chest and abdomen. From Figure 2-1 you can see that these so-called milk ridges are paired and extend from high on the chest wall to the groin. Later, paired milk glands appear along these ridges. In the cat and dog we find six or seven paired glands developing. A similar arrangement is also found in the pig, the rabbit and a wide variety of other mammals. Some mammals show a lack of development of the complete milk ridge with milk glands developing only on the chest or only on the abdomen. Paired mammary glands are found only in the abdominal region in the cow, the goat, the whale and the lion. Single paired milk glands evolve in the pectoral or chest area in such

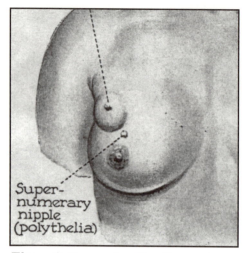

Fig. 2-2. A Rudimentary Nipple can develop along the milk ridge.

Super-numerary nipple (polythelia)

animals as the elephant, the walrus, and members of the ape family.

The milk ridges that unfold in the human fetus gradually fade long before birth, leaving a pair of budding mammary glands on the pectoral or chest area. Occasionally the milk ridge persists in a rudimentary form along the lower chest and even on the abdomen. This gives rise to undeveloped nipples and, rarely, even functioning breast tissue. Hence, one may discover an incidental atrophic nipple in the lower chest or upper abdomen in a man or woman, that is, for the most part, of little consequence. See Figure 2-2.

Among the family of mammals, breast cancer is found most often in the human. It very rarely occurs spontaneously in the rat and dog; but it is found in no other mammalian creature. Through chemicals and breeding, breast cancer can be produced in the laboratory rat; and in this way cancer can be studied.

Glandular Structure

The breast is divided into 15 to 20 lobes, radially positioned

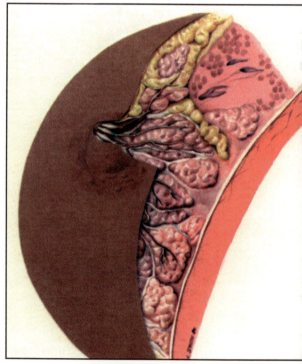

Fig. 2-3. Glandular structure showing the lobes and ducts. Most cancer originate in the ducts.

Where it All Begins

about the nipple as seen in Figure 2-3. These lobes in turn are sectioned into lobules which in turn are formed by hundreds of acini, which are the basic units that secrete milk. Channels that drain the acini, lobules and lobes converge at the nipple as ducts. Each duct has its own separate set of lobes, lobules and acini; and a copious layer of fat separates the lobules and surrounds the developing breast tissue.

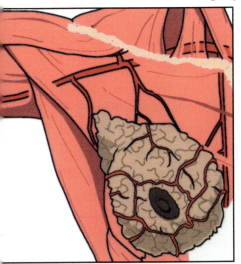

Fig. 2-4. The Arteries of the Breast. Under the influence of female hormones the blood supply increases.

Blood and Lymphatic Supply

A maze of blood vessels feeds into the breast tissue. See Figure 2-4. Estrogen hormones from the ovary regulate circulation to the breast by dilating the arteries and veins. These blood vessels, especially veins, serve as pathways for cancer spread and evidence suggests that cancer is already seeding into the circulation long before the primary tumor can be palpated. However, if the body is not overwhelmed, the immune system is able to destroy these early malignant cells.

Another important network that provides channels for cancer spread is the lymphatic system seen in Figure 2-5. The lymphatic vessels are much like veins but so thin-walled that they are generally invisible to the naked eye. Consequently, one may tend to forget their importance.

But in our anatomical road map these lymph channels are the major route allowing cancer cells to spread into deeper structures called lymph nodes. Therefore we must have a clear idea where these lymph nodes are located and be able to examine them for enlargement and tenderness. The lymph nodes that drain the breast are clustered, for the most part, in the axilla, or armpit. One must carefully palpate the axilla along with the breast for suspicious irregularities and tenderness.

The lymph channels ordinarily contain a clear fluid, that is nothing more than blood without the red blood cells. They are as plentiful as the capillaries and represent a vital part of the circulation. Blood, except for the red cells, seeps into these lymph channels and eventually this circulatory fluid

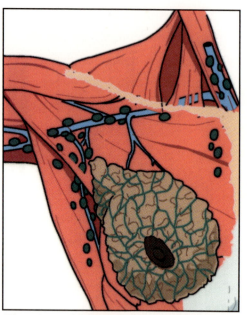

Fig. 2-5. Veins and Lymphatics. Veins and lymph channels (in green) are laced throughout the breast and axilla (armpit). Lymph channels drain into the lymph nodes which connect to the blood stream. The lymph channels and veins are the main routes by which cancer spreads.

is strained by lymph nodes, and eventually is returned to the general circulation. The lymph nodes are an important link in our defense system against cancer spread and cancer cells are trapped in the lymph nodes where many are destroyed. But some cells eventually escape the lymph nodes and are carried further until finally they empty into the general circulation and are then carried to such places as the lungs, liver and brain.

As mentioned above, the majority of lymph nodes that drain the breast are found nestled in the armpit; and consequently, the major flow of cancer cells from the breast by way of the lymphatics is laterally towards the axilla (armpit). It is this group of nodes that you and your physician will be carefully checking for enlargement and tenderness. Any non-tender mass in the breast with a firm nodule in the axilla demands immediate investigation for cancer.

However, lymph nodes in the axilla may also be enlarged and painful if there is infection in the breast or local infection in the axilla, or even in the arm or distal hand. A common occurrence is a minor skin infection in a hair follicle in the armpit with an associated enlarged node.

Muscles Under the Breast

There are two important muscles underlying the breast: The pectoralis major and the pectoralis minor noted in Figure 2-6. They are significant because cancer cells can migrate directly into the muscle tissue or travel by way of lymphatic channels to lymph nodes that lie between the muscles.

The pectoralis major lies immediately under the breast and fat layer. It originates along the margin of the sternum (breast bone) medially and clavicle (collar bone) above. A few slips spring from the rib cage below. The muscle then sweeps laterally across the chest wall to insert as a fibrous band into the humerus (arm bone) tucked under the deltoid shoulder muscle.

The pectoralis achieves its greatest development in the bird family where it becomes the highly specialized, powerful muscle of flight.

If this muscle is removed during cancer surgery it may cause only slight functional impairment. However, the deformity is very significant.

The pectoralis minor is a much smaller muscle that lies beneath the pectoralis major. It helps to stabilize the shoulder in concert with other muscles and if surgically removed there is no appreciable loss of function; but again, it adds to the deformity.

The mutilation of radical surgery

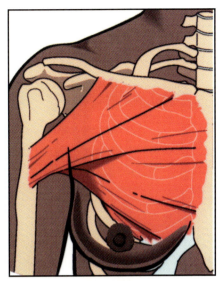

Fig. 2-6. Muscles under the Breast. The muscles under the breast are almost never removed as was done with the Halstead radical surgery. The standard modified radical mastectomy does not require removal of the muscles.

with removal of the pectoralis muscles has been replaced by more conservative procedures. If the cancer is discovered in time, in many instances the breast need not be removed. Only the cancer itself is excised along with some lymph nodes from the armpit.

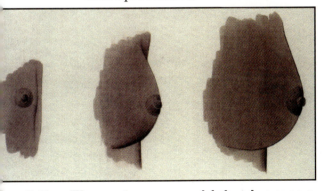

ig. 2-7. The estrogens which increase harply at puberty with the maturation of e ovaries are responsible for the begin-ing of menstruation and breast develop-ent.

Hormone Control of Human Breast Tissue

At birth the male and female breasts are essentially the same. The nipples are inverted and the surrounding coin-shaped skin, the areola, is slightly pigmented. Then a few days after birth, the areola darkens, nipples evert and the breast tissue swells in about 70 percent of newborns. Half of these babies will then secrete a cloudy fluid called 'witch's milk'. These changes are due to the influence of estrogen flowing into the child from the mother's blood stream by way of the placenta. But in two to three weeks after birth these changes will subside and the child's breast will ease into a resting stage. Breast tissue in both sexes will remain in a similar state of repose for years—until the awakening at puberty.

As puberty dawns, about age ten to twelve, all sorts of transformations begin to take place. Little children begin sprouting like weeds. Acne starts popping out. Little boys' voices start crackling and deepening into maturity. Pubic and axillary hair growth and muscular development are a part of this process. Little girls begin to snicker and talk about *boys*; and boys start looking at budding girls in a different way. Dating and dancing and going steady are a normal progression.

Ovaries have matured to the point that they can respond to the follicle stimulating hormone (FSH) produced by the pituitary gland located at the base of the brain. From the diagram in Figure 2-8, you can see that FSH hormone induces the ovary to form follicles which in turn produce estrogens. As the estrogen level rises even higher in the early teen years, ovaries begin to produce eggs, and the menstrual cycle begins. The estrogens are responsible for all the female characteristics, such as the high pitched voice, distribution of fat, shape of the pelvis, the smooth face, and, of course, the maturation of the breast.

In the pre-teen years enough estrogens cause a swelling under the nipple called the prepubertal bud. As the breast begins to protrude, glandular tissue spreads out in a fairly uniform circular manner and in a few short years the general contour of the young adult female breast is attained. See Figure 8.

During the first three to seven days of the menstrual cycle there is vaginal bleeding, or active menstrual flow as depicted in Figure 2-8. This corresponds to a temporary low level of estrogen production. When estrogen is at a low level, the lining of the uterus or womb cannot be maintained and it is shed in the form of menstrual flow.

About the seventh day of the cycle, new levels of estrogen are gradually being secreted by the ovary under the influence of the FSH from

Where it All Begins

the pituitary gland.

When the estrogen blood level reaches a certain point the lining of the uterus can be maintained and menstruation ceases. The lining continues to thicken for the next seven to ten days. The estrogen buildup also

Fig. 2-8. Female Hormones. The menstrual cycle averages 28 days. During the first half of the cycle estrogen causes a build up of the lining of the womb. The lining is then thickened and develops more blood vessels as the result of progesterone. When the production of these female hormones decreases, menstruation takes place. During the latter part of the cycle just before menstruation, the breast has enlarged by 50 per cent under the influence of these hormones. It is believed that estrogen is a factor in the development of breast cancer.

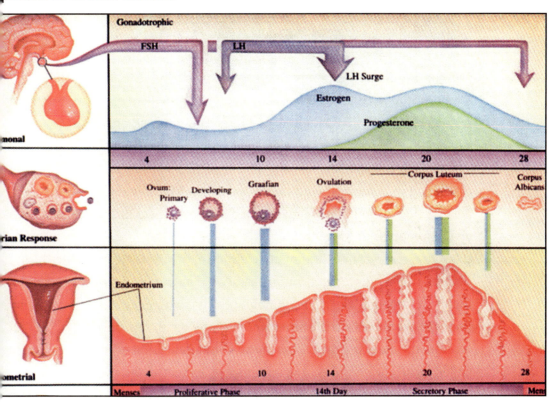

affects the breasts. There is a 50 percent increase in volume. The breasts become firm and occasionally tender. At this stage a tumor or cancer may be easily missed during physical examination. That's why your doctor will tell you to *examine your breasts a few days after the menstrual period ceases.*

About the fourteenth day, or mid-cycle, the follicle produces an egg which travels by way of the Fallopian tube to the lining of the uterus already prepared by estrogen stimulation. Refer to Figure 2-8. At the same time the high level of estrogen inhibits the flow of FSH from the pituitary and stimulates the pituitary gland to secrete the luteinizing hormone (LH) which acts on the ruptured follicle to produce progesterone. Progesterone is needed to further develop the lining of the uterus to make it hospitable and able to nourish the egg should it become impregnated. Towards the end of the cycle the rising tide of progesterone inhibits the LH from the pituitary which in turn causes a fall of progesterone.

By this time both progesterone and estrogen are at a low ebb and the uterine lining can no longer be maintained. Consequently menstrual flow begins anew as the lining of the uterus is shed.

Should pregnancy take place, the ovaries continue to supply the estrogen hormone in even larger volume and one of the major target organs, the breast, responds by growth and elaboration of the lobes and lobules. There is marked engorgement and enlargement of 2 to 3 times the resting state and pigmentation of the areola deepens and spreads to the adjacent breast skin. Veins dilate and stretch marks appear. After delivery and cessation of pregnancy, the hormone prolactin is released from the pituitary and combined with the action of a suckling baby, the breast produces a flow of milk that is maintained so long as suckling continues, even up to 36 months or longer. After milk production has ended, the breast proceeds to a resting state. Following childbirth, breast tissue is less dense and cancers can be discovered more readily by palpation. If a breast mass is found during pregnancy, mammography is sometimes delayed until the final month or so of the pregnancy. Ultrasound can be used to detect whether the mass is a cyst. There is no contraindication of removing a mass under local anesthesia during pregnancy. In fact if the mass is a cancer, definitive surgery may be carried out in spite of the pregnancy. The baby is not affected.

At the time of the menopause, in response to further lowering of estrogen, the breast atrophies and is replaced by fat. The contour becomes even more lax and small cancers can then be more easily palpated and seen on x-ray.

"Now then, are there any questions or comments before we show the movie on breast cancer detection? Yes young man, what is your question?"

A tall gangling youth awkwardly stood up in the back of the room and asked, "What about men? Do men get breast cancer too?"

After the giggling died down (teenagers laugh about almost anything) I spoke. "What's your name?"

"Amos Wilson."

"Yes Amos, it's true. Men do get breast cancer, but it is extremely rare. It's so rare that most of the time no one thinks that a sore or lump in the male breast is a cancer until it has spread and is probably incurable. So men must also be on the lookout for themselves as well as the women in their lives.

"But the most common cancer today in black men is lung cancer and almost all of it can be prevented by not smoking. You don't smoke do you Amos?"

Amos smiled and, of course, the teenagers snickered.

———

"Thank you everyone for your attention. This overview that I've presented is intended to answer some basic questions about the structure and function of the breast. I hope that it will also serve as a focal point for additional questions that you may wish to discuss at home or with your family doctor. You know, if you have a better understanding of where breast cancer begins, you should be able to appreciate your role in detecting breast cancer and warning others of the danger signals."

There has been a proliferation of breast cancer survivor organizations since the early 1990s. These groups have emerged to empower women and to provide a clarion voice to speak to their demands and point of view. For black women, it was not long before they realized that their needs could not be adequately addressed by a Caucasian dominated organization. Certainly the guidance of the Susan G Komen Fund, the American Cancer Society, The National Breast Cancer Coalition, and other organizations were absolutely vital to survival and growth, but the nurturing at the local level had to come from the innate black cultural and social structure.

When breast cancer survivors get together to share coping strategies their lives are enhanced, their focus is sharpened, and their energies are combined and directed. There is also some evidence that social ties and support networks increase longevity more so for black breast cancer survivors than their white counterparts.

Reynolds P Boyd PT Roberts S et al: The relationship between social ties and survival among black and white breast cancer patients;Can Epidem Biomarkers and Prevention vol 3 253-259 Apr/May 1994

CHAPTER THREE

A CASE FOR SHERLOCK HOLMES
Making the Diagnosis

for a hundred years we've observed and admired Sherlock Holmes as he deciphered baffling mysteries with his unique brand of expertise. The detective would methodically sift the clues and meticulously dissect each case using his fine sense of inductive reasoning. What seemed at first glance to be a string of disconnected facts would be dramatically interwoven into a pattern of logic and order. Ultimately, to our utter astonishment, Holmes would take us through the maze of clues that eventually pointed to the guilty party. His assistant, the befuddled Dr Watson, would finally raise his eyebrow and exclaim, "By jove Holmes, you're right".

In the same way the fictional character, Sherlock Holmes, demonstrated his talent for solving mysteries, health workers and patients in the real world must pool their talent and determination to solve the breast cancer mystery that confronted over 150,000 newly diagnosed women in 1990, and another 183,000 new cases in 1993. In 1996 the toll soared to 185,700 new cases of breast cancer.[26]

Indeed, the pursuit, the diagnosis, and the treatment of breast cancer is medical detective work of a high order. Many characters are involved and all play an essential part—research workers, physicians, hospital personnel, ministers, and the patient herself.

It can not be emphasized enough that every woman must assume full partnership in detecting breast cancer. This means awareness and knowing the warning signs. This is absolutely crucial in detecting the breast cancer villain before irretrievable damage is done. The doctor's training and the tools of medicine can only work effectively when the cancer criminal is not ignored or sheltered, but promptly exposed for effective elimination.

It has been reported that more than 90 percent of breast cancers are detected by the patient (this figure may be decreasing with increased use of routine mammography).1 In some cases a minor injury may prompt a woman to examine the breast and thus discover the lump. The problem is that these tumors are often reported after the cancer has spread. The National Cancer Institute survey in 1971 reported that in 68 percent of new cases among black women, breast cancer had already metastasized when first diagnosed; however, in only 58 percent of white women had the spread of cancer already occurred when first seen.2 There is no question that the chance for cure decreases precipitously if there is obvious spread at the time of first discovery. Cure rate for cancer confined to the breast should be 80 percent or more. This excellent prognosis quickly falls to a 25 to 50 percent survival if the cancer has metastasized when first uncovered.

Consequently, beginning about age twenty, every young woman should begin the habit of checking her breasts monthly to detect unusual nodules.3

BREAST SELF EXAMINATION

Early diagnosis is the goal of Breast Self-Examination (BSE) spearheaded by the American Cancer Society. Studies have suggested that regular BSE, a simple maneuver to master, can actually save lives.3 This, however, has been disputed in some quarters. A physician or other trained health provider can guide you through the various steps as you learn to examine your own breast. Also there are instructive brochures provided without charge at all American Cancer Society Units across the country. Although the exact procedure proposed may vary somewhat among physicians, the general principles are the same. One should systematically search the breast for lumps or thickening on a monthly basis. This should be done about ten days after the menstrual flow begins each and every month. If there is no menstruation because of surgery or menopause then an exam on the same day each month is adequate. The examination is divided between inspection and palpation. See Figure 3-1.

Inspection: Stand before the mirror, chest exposed, and inspect the breasts looking for obvious deformity or irregularity. Notice superficial vein engorgement, skin dimpling or discoloration, or rash over the nipple area. Now lean forward. Again look in the mirror with a good light. Do both breasts move away from the chest wall in a similar manner or is there

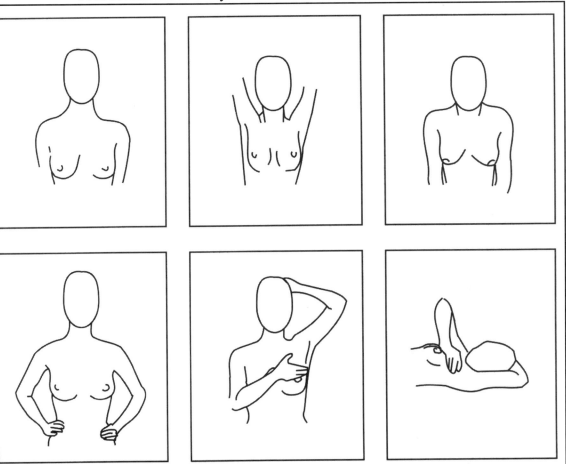

Fig. 3-1. Breast Self Examination (BSE). Monthly BSE beginning at age 20 should continue on a regular basis for a lifetime. It is especially important for young black women since they have breast cancer at twice the rate of white women before age 40. The heightened mortality rate in black women is even more significant.

restrictions or dimpling not noticed before? Does either nipple appear to be pulled to one side or the other?

Palpation: The entire breast and arm pit should be palpated systematically section by section. It is necessary for each woman to become familiar with the many soft nodules normally present in her breast, because everyone is different. It is best to use the flattened hand and the flat of the fingers rather than the curled finger tips; and it helps to steady the tissue with your other hand as you compress the breast against the chest wall. I prefer to have the patient examine herself methodically while lying down, beginning in the armpit pressing the breast tissue against the chest wall section by section searching for a dominant mass. Imagine a small lump of cauliflower under a folded bath towel. That's just about what you're feeling for—an irregular firm mass that is not tender. Occasionally it may be odd shaped and hurt when compressed. After checking the breast, one section at a time, and finding no dominant lump(s), you should gently compress the nipple between thumb and forefinger for evidence of blood or discharge. Thirty percent of women over the age of 60 with nipple discharge and no breast lump eventually prove to have breast cancer.

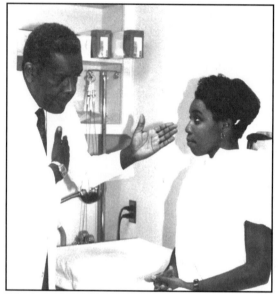

Fig. 3-2. Professional instruction and examination should occur on a yearly basis. More than half of cancers found in black women have already spread when first discovered.

With monthly BSE you will soon know your normal nodularity and lumpiness. If there is any question, by all means, have your doctor go over it with you. Most breast lumps are either normal or represent benign disease. The chance of a lump being cancer increases with advancing years. Therefore, breast self examination is every bit as crucial as any detective insight your doctor can bring to bear on the case. According to the American Cancer Society only 25 percent of black women examine their breasts on a regular monthly basis. If breast cancer mortality is to be challenged successfully, not only must you engage in BSE regularly each month, but you must take it upon yourself to encourage all of your adult women friends to do likewise.

Periodically it is important to allow a physician or other trained health provider to examine the breast with you. Your questions and concerns should be discussed at that time. A yearly examination would seem adequate, and more frequent exams are warranted if a woman has certain risk factors.

DIFFERENTIAL DIAGNOSIS

Once the breast lump is known to be present, the capable detective, like any worthy Sherlock Holmes, regards the mass as a prime suspect. The evidence must be tested, and conclusions drawn. Is this lump a cancer, a cyst or some benign interloper? What is the correct diagnosis among all the possibilities? Across the board only one in eight breast masses is actually a cancer. This figure rises sharply in the older age groups. After age 50, all breast lumps must be considered malignant until proven otherwise.

If the lump is not a cancer, what are the other possibilities? Several benign tumors come to mind. Your doctor will consider fibrocystic dysplasia, fibroadenoma, ductal papilloma, and fat necrosis. Let's briefly examine two of the more common benign problems that can be confused with cancer.

Fibrocystic Dysplasia

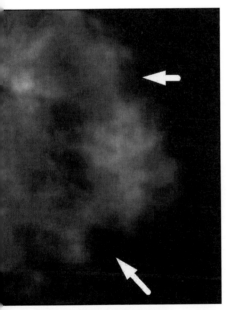

The most common tumor found in the breast between age 35 and the menopause is fibrocystic dysplasia, also called fibrocystic disease.[4] It manifests itself before the menopause as multiple nodules in both breasts. A single nodule may be quite prominent and the rest very small or not palpable. It may be impossible to distinguish fibrocystic dysplasia from cancer and require aspiration, mammography (x-ray examination), needle biopsy, and perhaps open biopsy to make the diagnosis.

After the menopause, estrogen hormone levels fall and fibrocystic dysplasia tends to soften and subside. Seldom does it cause significant discomfort, although occasionally the breasts may become taut and tender just before menstruation. A well-fitting brassiere can reduce the discomfort. If the discomfort of fibrocystic dysplasia is not controlled by aspirin or other simple

Fig. 3-3. The multiple dark round areas reveal fibrocystic dysplasia.

analgesics, then avoiding certain foods and medications that contain methylxanthine such as chocolate and certain asthma medications, is usually beneficial.

Methylxanthine is also found in coffee, tea, Anacin, Dristan, Midol and other medications commonly used. As a last resort, if the breast dis-

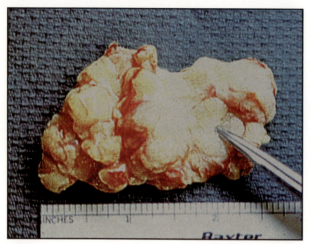

Fig. 3-4. Biopsy of Fibrocystic Dysplasia. Only with microscopic examination can this be distinguished from cancer.

comfort is unremitting, Vitamin E and androgen hormones can be used with good relief.**5** Most of the nodularity will disappear. If a dominant lump persists, then biopsy is imperative regardless of mammographic results.**6** Also it should be noted that since nicotine stimulates cystic formation, smoking cigarettes may contribute to fibrocystic dysplasia.

It is widely accepted that women with fibrocystic dysplasia have an increased risk of developing breast cancer, though studies from England have challenged this view.**7,8**

Although most of these benign nodules are solid and discrete some are connected with neighboring nodules and some become cystic and fill with fluid. A diagnostic office procedure, transillumination, may be suggested by your doctor to show if the tumor is solid or cystic. It is quite probable that the medical detective will prefer a needle aspiration of the lump with the skin anesthetized. Many times a thin fluid, straw colored or pale greenish-gray, will be removed and the mass eliminated forever. The fluid is checked for cancer cells. If negative, the breast is simply observed for several months for possible recurrence of the cyst. If aspiration does not deflate the nodule it is assumed to be solid and if it is enlarging and fairly distinct from the other masses, a biopsy is mandatory to rule out cancer even if the mammogram does not suggest malignancy. It is true that the vast majority of cystic lesions tend to be benign and indeed 90 percent are successfully handled by aspiration. If there is a recurrence of the same cyst after a second aspiration, I

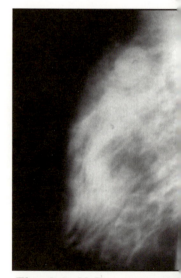

Fig. 3-5. X-Ray reveals round mass, most like a fibroadenoma in th upper part of the breas

A Case for Sherlock Holmes

would recommend surgical excision of the cyst even if the aspirate is negative for cancer cells.

If a woman is known to have fibrocystic dysplasia, it is imperative that breast self examination be done monthly about ten days after the menstrual period begins. A physician or other professional should examine the breast every six to eight months and a record kept for follow-up.

Fibroadenoma

This is a benign tumor that can only be distinguished from a cancer by microscopic examination.[9] It usually presents as a single lesion,

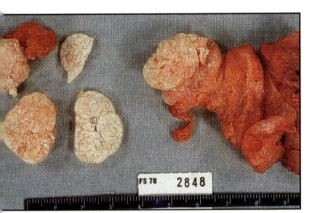

Fig. 3-6. Biopsy of Fibroadenoma. Note the sharp borders of this benign tumor found most often in young women. There increased risk of cancer in these cases.

although, a number of these growths can arise in the breast simultaneously. The mass is a freely movable tumor that is non-tender, and when first discovered, ranges in size from a peanut to a walnut. Some believe that estrogen stimulation is somehow causative, because it grows rapidly during pregnancy when estrogen level is high; and birth control pills stimulate the rapid growth of fibroadenoma. It almost always develops in young women—late teens or early twenties; in fact, it is the number one breast tumor by a wide margin under age twenty-five. If you happen to be in that age bracket with a breast tumor, your doctor may give you reassurance that it is simply a benign tumor. His judgement is based on your age. He cannot be sure by physical examination although in the face of a negative mammogram the diagnosis will probably be correct. After years of detecting these lumps I must admit I've hazard a diagnosis like most surgeons. But I've always insisted that all such tumors be removed to definitely rule out cancer.

Many years ago a 26-year-old black mother of two came to my office for a second opinion about a lump in her breast. Yes, it was there, about as big as the end of your thumb. Freely movable, no pain. Mammogram showed the tumor without any distinct cancer markings.

"What did your doctor tell you?," I asked.

"Said it was a tumor, that was probably not a bad one, that I should have it out. What do you think, Doctor Johnson? I don't want to be experimented on if it is nothing to worry about."

"Well, I suppose your doctor wants it out just to be sure. Your mammogram was not diagnostic for cancer, and the chances are good that it is a benign tumor. However, we cannot be completely sure unless we check it under the microsope. I would have to agree with your doctor. Have it removed right away to be sure."

The young woman put off surgical removal of the lump. She wanted to wait and get another opinion. I saw her about a year or so later. She wanted me to check the lump. Sure enough the tumor was much larger and seemed to be fixed to the underlying muscle. Enlarged lymph nodes were easily felt in the armpit. She had not gotten another medical opinion after all, and had only confided in friends. Now, there was pain. The growing tumor had been ignored as long as possible. Now she was forced to come to grips with the specter of cancer. Like so many other black women, young and old, she had allowed a malignancy to grow and spread. Two years later the cancer thief robbed another young family in spite of surgery, radiation and all the rest.

In real life Sherlock Holmes doesn't always win. The lesson to be learned is that regardless of your age, if a lump is felt in the breast do not delay seeking and accepting competent medical attention. Remember, only early cancer promptly treated is curable in more than 80 percent of cases.

Mastodynia

Mastodynia, or painful breast(s), is seldom the first sign of cancer. However, it must be thoroughly evaluated to be certain that an underlying cancer is not the culprit. Careful physical examination and mammography are essential. Fibrocystic disease is commonly painful and tender before mensturation. If cancer is not present and pain is disabling and not amenable to bra support, or common analgesics, then other measures should be tried. Physicians may suggest that all hormonal therapy be halted including menopause medication and birth control pills. If blood tests reveal that prolactin levels are elevated, bromocriptine may be introduced. In resistant cases Danazol has had good success. Also some women have responded to diuretics, or tamoxifen.

DIAGNOSTIC TOOLS [Sifting the Clues]

Mammography (X-ray Examination)

Along with BSE and periodic examinations by the health provider, mammography (x-ray) examination of the breast has proven to be the most valuable tool for the medical detective.**10**

With the proliferation of mammography screening centers it is important that the quality of the examinations be superior. If the center you choose is sanctioned by the American College of Radiology then you can be certain that it meets the highest standards and the report will be as accurate as possible.

In February, 1993 the feasibility of early mammography was raised. Data was presented at a National Cancer Institute conference that indicated that screening mammography before age 50 did not reduce breast cancer death rate in women ages 40 to 49.**21**

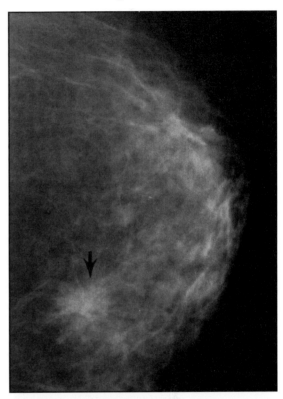

Fig3-7A. Mammograaam with a suspicious lesion noted by the arrow. A needle biopsy revealed cancer.

Therefore some suggested that it was not cost effective to screen before age 50. However, the American College of Radiology, the American Cancer Society, and other groups stated that the study was flawed; and they continued to recommend screening at least every two years from age 40 to 50 and then every year from age 50. In 1996, the American Cancer Society (ACS), according to Dr Robert Smith, head of the Department of Detection and Treatment of the ACS in Atlanta, advocated yearly screening, beginning at age 40 (instead of every 2 years).

In my opinion, screening for the general population should begin at age 35 to make an impact on the 40 to 49 year old group. In fact I believe that black women should be screened on a yearly basis from age 30, because the rate of cancer is one and a half times that of whites before age 35.[33] Breast cancer not only occurs earlier in black women, but it is more aggressive and spreads sooner. Young black women are more likely to present with advanced disease, simply because it was not discovered in time. Although the incidence of breast cancer in sub-Sahara Africa is only a fraction of that in western countries, a large proportion of breast cancer in black Africans occurs in the below 30 age group. For example 6.4 percent of breast cancers in Sudan and 14.7 percent of breast cancers in Nigeria occur before the 30th birthday.[31,32] There is no proof that Breast Self - Examination impacts on mortality, but there is enough evidence to

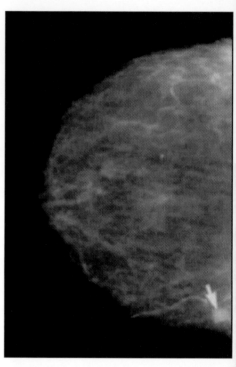

Fig3-7B. Mammogram showing a fatty breast in an older woman. Cancer is fairly easy to observe.

bolster a belief that it does indeed reduce mortality. The same can be said for Pap smear screening and other screenings that we believe make a difference.The need for early mammogram screening in black women has not been proven by any prospective inquiry. Nevertheless there is enough evidence to support this notion. See Chapter 6, page 94, *Starting Mammography at 30 Something.*

The official screening guidelines purported by our leading cancer organizations remain in a state of confusion. In 1996, for example, the National Cancer Institute's Dr John Gohagan, chief of the early detection branch, declared that it was no longer in the business of recommending any age to start mammogram screening.

Prostate cancer screening is regularly done in black men ten years younger than white men, simply because it occurs earlier in black men and the cancer is more aggressive and spreads early on. The same reasoning should be acceptable for breast cancer screening in black women.

We encourage Pap smear screening every 2-3 years for cervical cancer starting at age 20, and then every year after age 30. Nobody frowns at that suggestion. But the incidence of cervical cancer is only a fraction of breast cancer at age 30 and the death rate is a third of the breast cancer death rate. Shouldn't we be consistent in screening for breast cancer which is more prevalent and dangerous than cervical cancer at age 30?

Mammography is still the best tool available for early detection, although it is by no means foolproof. From 10 to 15 percent of cancers will

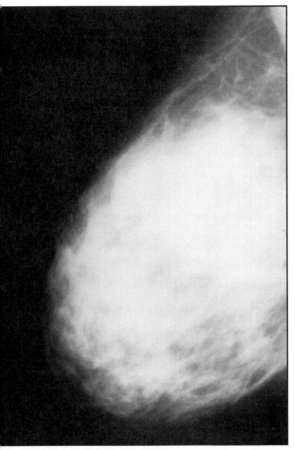

g. 3-7C. Mammogram of a young oman with dense breasts. Cancer may e missed in 15% of such cases.

be missed by mammography due to the breast density, faulty equipment, and misinterpretation by the radiologist. In many centers errors by the physician are reduced by double reading. It has been demonstrated that an additional 5-15 percent of cancers are detected if mammogram x-rays are read by a second radiologist.[27,28]

Even though mammography is our principle means of early diagnosis, black women must take it upon themselves to insist that their physicians order the test. A study by Columbia University School of Public Heath reported that physicians' recommendations for mammography were different according to race. If a physician had a predominantly black practice, mammography screening was recommended only 7 percent of the time compared to the physician with a white practice where mammography was offered 23% of the time.[30]

Breast x-ray was first tried in the late 1940's. In those days machines were crude and radiation exposure was high. There was little enthusiasm for mammography early on and the technique lay fallow until the early 1960's, when investigators devised x-ray machines dedicated exclusively to x-raying the breast. Mammography first became available for a large population during a wide scale screening project sponsored by the New York Health Insurance Program, commonly called the HIP project. A modified x-ray machine had been developed that resulted in less radiation exposure and better defined negatives.[11] See Chapter 6, page 85.

Mammography continued to evolve along several pathways with improvement in the radiation-producing apparatus and changes in the material upon which the image was recorded. In the early 1960's the French were developing an x-ray machine that used, instead of tungsten, molybdenum as a target for the x-rays. They also placed the anode closer to the target and found that these changes produced better definition in their images. In 1970 these alterations had been incorporated into a tidy efficient x-ray unit called the Senograph and marketed in the United States. It replaced the old tungsten x-ray model of the early 1960's. This new Senograph quite clearly detected very early cancers that could not be palpated.

Micro-calcifications and minute breast patterns indicative of malignancy were readily detected. There was also further reduction in radiation exposure with the new equipment from the 7 to 15 rads down to 2.5 rads.

About that time Dr John Wolfe reported on his experience in the development of xeroradiography (1968). The image was not recovered on a negative film as in the Senograph. It was imaged on a paper as a positive rendition. As a result, we now had two reliable and efficient methods widely available to uncover breast cancer before it could be palpated.

Nevertheless there was some question as to which was the better medium to view the mammogram, the celluloid film negative or the positive image on paper produced by the xeroradiograph. In the early days some technicians in training, and those at screening clinics preferred the xerograms. But many trained radiologists accustomed to looking at negatives found that interpreting the negative film was satisfactory and in some cases preferable. The Xerox process allowed for little error in exposure and often repeat films were required. In 1992 the Xerox Corporation, the manufacturer of xeroradiograph paper announced that it would no longer produce that material since there was little demand for the product. At that point the celluloid film became, and continues to be the standard of care.

When hundreds and even thousands of women are being screened, use of the 105 mm roll Senograph film has definite advantages in being less expensive and requiring less time per patient. The roll of Senograph film can be examined at the end of the screening day thus lessening time of the patient in the screening center, sometimes by as much as 20 minutes. With improvement in film, screens, etc., the radiation exposure using the Senograph is now in the range of 0.2 to 0.3 rad, compared to 2 or 3 rads in xerograms. These are extremely low doses and the induction of breast cancer or other cancers by radiation is now of little or no significance after the age of 40.[35] Even so, scientists are working on even more sophisticated equipment with xonics. This method will use electrons instead of photons to form the x-ray beam. They will produce images on Mylar instead of paper or celluloid and exposure will be reduced to only 0.05 to 0.1 rad.

Dr Wolfe found another use for mammography.[12] He theorized that cancer was very unlikely if certain patterns were found on the mammogram. Other workers corroborated these findings.[13] The breast patterns reflecting a high density and cord structure and ductal hypertrophy developed cancer in 5 percent of the cases. The chance of developing cancer in a breast of low density and sparse tissue was only 0.5 percent. In either case the malignancy developed within three years. Other specialists, however, have remained skeptical and today, by and large, films with differing patterns are not often used to predict the chance of cancer development.

Digital Mammography

Since 1996 the cutting edge of technology is the computerized technique that enhances the mammogram with an infinite scale of gray tones that improves contrast. This new digitization vastly enhances mammography in dense breasts and allows computer aided diagnosis with enhanced image interpretation. It also allows for telemammography, that is, transmission by modem to distant sites for specialist examination. This research is being pursued by an umbrella organization: The National Digital Mammography Development Group. Various components are based in many medical centers around the country including the University of North Carolina, the University of Chicago, General Electric R&D System, etc.

Thermography

The tools of the medical Sherlock Holmes do not stop with digital mammography and its various developments. Also available is thermography.14 There is some controversy regarding its usefulness, although some physicians find it helpful. This device is a heat sensor apparatus that is

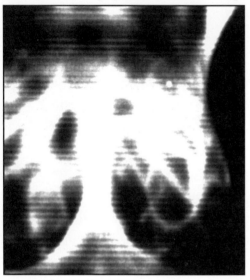

Fig. 3-8. Normal Thermogram of left breast.

designed to record differences in temperature throughout the breast onto a permanent record. Malignant breast lesions often have a higher temperature than normal breast tissue and some success has been noted in detecting early cancer that was otherwise obscure. Inflammatory disease and benign tumors can also register an increased temperature; and the method has been found to be fraught with frequent false negative and false positive findings. Consequently most centers do not rely on thermography for anything more than a confirmatory technique in the face of positive physical and/or mammographic findings.

Some screening centers noting a 20 percent false positive rate have omitted thermography altogether. Others still argue that thermography is of some benefit in the doubtful case. Occasional so-called false positive cases do indeed develop a breast cancer two to three years later. If the mammogram is equivocal and the physical examination is not definite, then a positive thermogram would be likely to prompt breast biopsy.

I have never personally ordered a thermography study for my patients. I just don't feel that the expense is justified. If a lump is suspicious on the mammogram, a biopsy must be done regardless of the results from the ther-

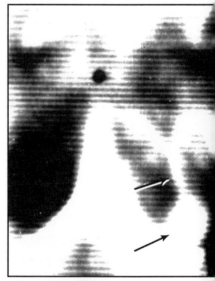

Fig. 3-9. Thermogram revea lesion in left breast.

mogram.

Thermography is defined by the American College of Radiology and American Thermographic Society as a "complimentary diagnostic tool that *may* be useful in the evaluation of breast disease when combined with both physical examination and mammography under the supervision of a qualified physician and a trained radiologist."

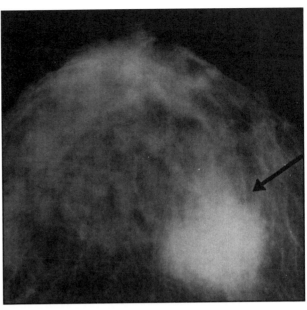

Fig. 3-10. Breast mass that may be solid or cystic.

Ultrasound

The ultrasound machine is a device that uses sound waves to distinguish solid masses from cysts. It operates on the principle that the density of cystic and solid structures reflect sound waves differently and thereby produce images that are easily differentiated. The accuracy in detecting cancer is only 60 to 75 percent. It finds its greatest usefulness in examining young women with dense breast tissue when a cyst is suspected.**15** New technology promises to improve the ultrasound ability to distinguish solid from cystic lesions. In 1997 the FDA is on the verge of approving the Ultramark 9, a high definition imaging system. This high definition ultrasound machine will greatly enhance our diagnostic ability and reduce the need for breast biopsy by 40 percent according to Dr Ellen Mendelson of the Western Pennsylvania Hospital in Pittsburgh.

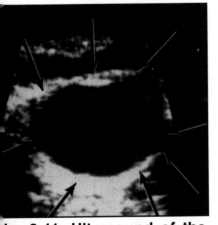

ig. 3-11. Ultrasound of the reast mass in Fig. 3-10 eveals that it is cystic and equires aspiration for further study.

Many surgeons, including myself, rely heavily on ultrasound to distinguish cystic and solid masses, so any improvement is welcome news. It is a good idea to insist on an ultrasound study before needle aspiration or biopsy of a breast lump.

Single Photon Emission Computed Tomography (SPECT)

This is an exciting new scanning device to detect breast cancer in young women, women with dense breasts, and high risk women. Dr David Preston at the Kansas University Medical Center has shown that SPECT is so sensitive that it can pick up breast cancer years before it is detected by mammography. *Mammography* detects cancer when the cancer tissue becomes more dense than the surrounding normal breast. *SPECT*, however, may show subtle architectural changes before change in density becomes a factor. Specifically, when a cancer begins to develop, it develops more estrogen receptor sites. When a patient is injected with radioactive estrogen (estradiol) it locks on to receptor sites in the new cancer. Then when the breast is scanned, the radioactive estrogen will be detected as it accumulates at the estrogen receptor locations. The technique is being evaluated and its role along with mammography is still being elucidated; however, I expect SPECT will become a major tool in early detection of the breast cancer villain, especially in young women with dense breasts.

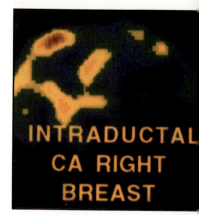

INTRADUCTAL CA RIGHT BREAST

Fig. 3-12. SPECT. With the next few years this w be extremely useful detecting breast cancer young women with den breast tissue. This is pa ticularly important young black women wi disproportionately mo breast cancer.

Diaphanography

This technique does not replace x-ray mammography, but may uncover very early cancers not detected by the mammogram. The principle use is to confirm what is found by other detecting methods. It involves transillumination with infra-red and photographing the result. The picture is then carefully examined for defects.16

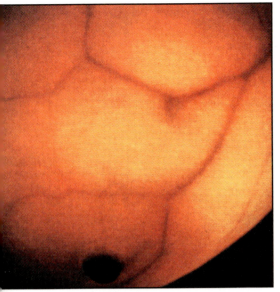 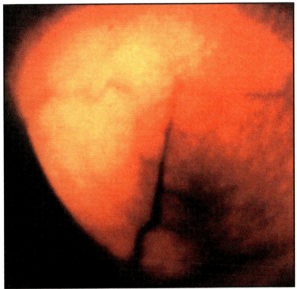

g. 3-13. Normal Right Diaphanogram. Fig. 3-14. Abnormal Left Diaphanogram.

Magnetic Resonance Imaging (MRI)

The MRI, so useful in neurological and orthopedic patient evaluation, does not have the same utility when it comes to uncovering breast cancer. Investigators have stated that the MRI fails to meet any of the four requirements for a successful screening modality. (1) Accessibility: These facilities are scarce and used primarily to detect bone and neurological defects. (2) Acceptability: Patient discomfort during a test is a deterrent. (3) Accuracy: The MRI will not detect small cancers. It will not detect micro-calcifications. It cannot reliably distinguish benign and malignant lesions. (4) Affordability: Because of the expense of equipment, prolonged time for handling and interpretation, the cost is very high and impractical for screening. At this juncture, MRI is not widely recommended for breast examination, and certainly not for breast cancer screening.[29]

However, a new form of MRI developed at Baylor University Medical Center may prove useful in detecting lobular carcinoma in situ (LCIS) which is not detectable with mammography. LCIS is a clear marker of impending breast cancer and this new MRI technique may be a breakthrough. The new technology is called, 3-D RODEO MRI (3-dimensional rotating delivery excitation off-resonance magnetic resonance imaging). It provides better contrast and 20 times higher resolution than regular MRI. A role in screening is being considered.

Nipple Discharge

Fluid discharging spontaneously from the nipple or provoked by gentle pressure may be either cloudy or blood tinged. The question of cancer, of course, is uppermost on the mind if one experiences blood or any fluid coming from the breast. In the majority of cases a benign lesion (papilloma) is the cause, but cancer is found with increasing frequency in older age groups.

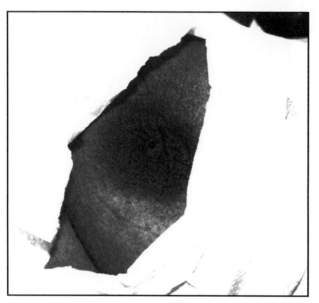

Breast cancers are associated with a bloody fluid discharge about 20 percent of the time even though a lump is not readily palpable. Therefore, careful detective work will mandate an x-ray exam and probably biopsy in the case of bloody discharge from the nipple.

On the other hand, a thin clear fluid discharge may be noted for years and be completely benign. If the discharge is copious and clear it may signal the presence of a prolactinoma tumor of the pituitary.

Fig. 3-15. Blood coming from the nipple. Breast cancers are associated with a bloody fluid discharge in about 20 per cent of the time, even though a lump is not readily palpable.

Aspiration of a Cyst

Aspiration finds its greatest use in young women with palpable masses that appear to be a cyst on mammography and ultrasound. The cysts may be deflated and the fluid checked for malignant cells. If the cyst disappears following drainage and the aspirate negative for cancer, no further intervention is required other than the routine periodic mammography, physical exams, and breast self-examination (BSE).

Biopsy

Whenever a mass or lump is located by palpation and/or mammography, etc., the next step is to obtain tissue for absolute identification. In many clinics the open breast biopsy is done on an out-patient basis under local anesthesia. However if the breast is pendulous or the lesion small and difficult to locate, the surgeon may elect to hospitalize the patient and do the open biopsy under general anesthesia with initial needle localization.

Many physicians prefer not to perform a mastectomy at the time of biopsy if the specimen is found to be cancerous. On the other hand some patients prefer immediate mastectomy if the biopsy is positive. I encourage postponing mastectomy following biopsy so that the tissue removed can be examined in greater detail after it is properly fixed and stained. That takes about two days. In the meantime, the patient and family can discuss the ramifications of various treatment options. It is not unusual for a patient to decide in favor of another treatment option even though mastectomy was the initial decision. So a short delay may have merit. According to a study done by Dr Fisher and his group, there is absolutely no adverse affect if mastectomy is delayed for two weeks after the biopsy.17

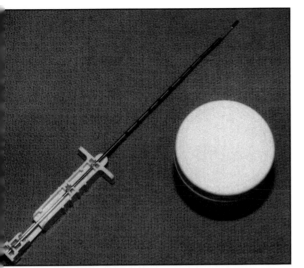

ig. 3-16A. Needle used with local anesesia to examine a suspicious breast sion. Open biopsy may be avoided.

Before submitting to the standard biopsy, you may wish to discuss the difference between aspiration cytology or core needle biopsy.

Core Needle Biopsy versus Aspiration Cytology

In lieu of open biopsy in which an incision is made over a breast lump and the lump extracted with the scalpel, a needle biopsy may be performed with obviously less invasion and trauma. The advantage of the needle approach is that a diagnosis may be obtained without leaving the telltale biopsy scar. Healing is rapid. There is no tissue distortion that may confuse the reading of future mammograms. There is no loss of time from work or general activity. And in these days of budgetary restraints, it is cost effective.

If the needle biopsy is positive, then certainly the patient is spared open biopsy and planning for definitive treatment may proceed forthwith.

If the needle biopsy is negative for cancer, and the lesion is suspicious because of family history, mammogram, ultrasound, or physical examination, then open biopsy, in my opinion, is mandatory. The open excisional biopsy remains the gold standard.

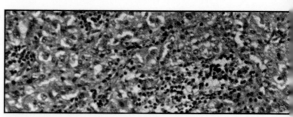

Fig. 3-16B. Cancer found on needle biopsy. An open biopsy for confirmation should be done as a preliminary step before mastectomy.

There are two methods of needle biopsy—Aspiration Cytology and Core Needle Biopsy. The least traumatic of the two is Aspiration Cytology, also called fine needle aspiration biopsy (FNAB). This procedure allows the physician to pass a very thin needle into a suspicious lesion under local anesthesia, to aspirate a small amount of tissue and fluid and quickly smear the material on a slide for microscopic examination. Usually 3 or 4 slides are made by the cytotechnician who is present at the procedure for immediate processing. The sensitivity and specificity are quite excellent and, when performed with skill and expertise, the procedure and results are highly acceptable by patient and physician. However, if the results are negative for cancer, even with a suspicious mammogram or physical findings, insist that confirmation of the results of FNAB be confirmed by excisional biopsy!

An alternative to Aspiration Cytology is Core Needle Biopsy with the Trucut needle (Baxter-Travenol). A needle of much greater caliber (18 guage to 14 gauge) than the FNAB is used to remove a core of tissue from the breast mass under local anesthesia. This method has the advantage of providing much more material for microscopic scrutiny. The cytotechnician need not be present, since immediate processing is not required. When properly performed, a definitive diagnosis is more likely with the Trucut core needle biopsy. Using the Ultrasound or other imaging device to guide the needle placement would improve efficacy and reduce the time of the procedure. However, should a tissue diagnosis be ambiguous, open biopsy would be the standard of care.

In February 1996, I was asked to review a case in which a breast cancer diagnosis was unduly delayed. The surgeon had performed a Trucut core biopsy of a breast mass which failed to show cancer. The pathology report indicated that there was no cancer in the small amount of tissue obtained. The report also suggested that the biopsy was inadequate. The doctor reassured the patient that cancer was not present. However, cancer was indeed present and when it was finally found three months later, by open biopsy, the cancer had advanced from a Stage I to a Stage II. Her chance for cure was reduced significantly.

Ask your doctor what the actual language of the biopsy report states. In this particular case the patient should have had an open biopsy, particularly with other risk factors being present. Previous biopsies had revealed precancerous lesions, and the woman's mother had had breast cancer.

But she was never advised that her previous biopsies were pre-malignant—only that they were negative. And not knowing that a negative needle biopsy in the face of important risk factors requires open biopsy, this black woman was misguided and the breast cancer diagnosis, to her detriment, was delayed. Unable to find a local physician to support her claim, my testimony based on standard guidelines found in the medical literature made the difference. She was awarded a judgement.

I suspect that Trucut core needle biopsies, properly performed, will replace the open biopsy in most instances of establishing a tissue diagnosis of breast lumps. In my view, Aspiration Cytology will be used less frequently, since it cannot distinguish a cancer that is infiltrating from a cancer that is not spreading.

Remember, though, if a core needle biopsy (Trucut) is equivocal, insist on the open excisional biopsy, especially if there are known risk factors present. Sherlock Holmes would insist on nothing less.

Stereotactic Core Needle Biopsy

For the non-palpable breast tumor that is seen on mammography, this new method of needle biopsy was developed.**34** The procedure is performed on a prone examination table with the breast suspended through an opening. Currently the Mammotome (Biopsys, Irvine, California) and the (Advanced Breast Biopsy Instrumentation) ABBI (United States Surgical, Norwalk, Connecticut) are the common technologies used in this country. Both systems are costly. The Mammotome is less invasive. The ABBI sys-

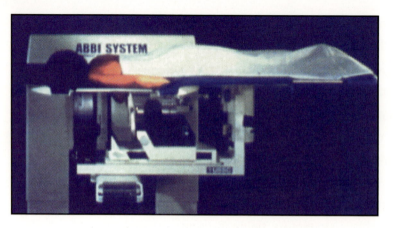

Fig. 3-17. The ABBI Table. A comfortable method of breast biopsy with minimal scar.

tem can remove up to a 20 mm tissue core and able to remove 50 times as much tissue. In 1997, Senator Edward Kennedy was leading the fight to be sure that the makers of the ABBI prove the efficacy and safety of the ABBI at 20 mm. It has already been approved at 3mm. Surgeons and radiologists believe that the diagnostic accuracy is very good; and, I suspect, that this technique will become the standard of care in selected cases.

Chest X-ray

The chest x-ray is one of the first clues to be examined in all cases of suspected breast cancer. Metastasis to the lung can be detected and if a solitary lesion found, surgical excision may be possible. If many lesions are present then proper chemotherapy or radiation should be used.

Bone Scan and Liver Scan

The bone scan is seldom done in the early and mid-stages of breast cancer. Unless there is bone pain or specific complaints the chance of finding a bone metastasis is less than 21 percent. On the other hand liver scan is worthwhile early on. It should be preceded by a much less expensive blood test. If the blood test is positive for some unidentified liver problem then the scan may be of assistance in diagnosing cancer.

Blood Tests

The alkaline phosphatase blood determination becomes elevated early in liver metastasis. Anywhere from 60-90 percent of those with breast cancer and liver spread will have an elevated result. However, all blood tests have limited value. The alkaline phosphatase can also be abnormal in a number of other unrelated conditions. A blood test to detect only cancer is not presently available. Of course it would be the ideal screening device and investigators are struggling to bring it into reality. Indeed, such a discovery would all but eliminate our prolonged detective endeavors.

Another important blood test requiring careful interpretation is the Carcino-embryonic Antigen (CEA).[18] This substance is elevated in about 50 percent of breast cancer patients. It is also observed in the blood of some patients with colon cancer and cancer of the pancreas. CEA may also be elevated in the case of liver cirrhosis, emphysema, peptic ulcer, and colitis. Nevertheless the CEA blood level should be checked if breast cancer is suspected. If cancer is later confirmed and adequately treated the CEA blood level should fall to normal in most cases. Any subsequent rise in the CEA may herald a recurrence of the malignancy even if there are no other clues. It has been noted that if the CEA level falls below 2.5 nanagrams following treatment (surgery or radiation) there is a 20 percent chance of recurrence in the ensuing two year period. If the CEA fails to fall below that point, the recurrence rate is 65 percent during the following two year post-treatment period.[19]

To corroborate the CEA results, several new markers (monoclonal antibodies) that signal tumor recurrence have been developed. The principal ones include: Cancer Associated Antigen (CA 15-3), Mucinoid Cancer Antigen (MCA), the Tissue Polypeptide Antigen (TPA), and Breast Cancer Antigen (BCA 225). Studies suggest that CA 15-3 is especially useful in corroborating the CEA test in detecting recurrent breast cancer ten months before any traces are detectable on physical or x-ray examination.

In 1995 a new tumor marker was reported called the CA 27-29 or Truquant Test. The sensitivity is 62 percent with an accuracy of 83 percent. It has been approved by the FDA and now in many cases is replacing the CA 15-3.[36] Nevertheless it must be emphasized that none of these tests are useful in screening for breast cancer, only for detecting recurrence.[22-24]

Prognostic Indicators

There are various observations and tests available that allow the doctor to gauge the severity of cancer in a particular patient. For example, a large cancer, attachment to the skin or chest wall and the presence of lymph nodes in the armpit, all signal a poor prognosis.

By determining the estrogen and progesterone receptor status of a cancer we can expect a correlation with rate of growth and chance of metastasis. Also, by observing the DNA behavior, the aggressiveness of a cancer can be predicted. Let us examine these prognostic indicators.

Estrogen Receptor and Progesterone Receptor (ER) (PR): In the early 1970's researchers at the University of Chicago and elsewhere gave us the Estrogen Receptor Theory. It has proven to be a device that has allowed us to direct hormone and chemotherapy to patients who may respond. Here's the way it operates. First, it was noted in 1959 that if an estrogen was labeled so you could follow it through the body, and it was injected into a laboratory animal, it would congregate in the ovary and breast tissue. It was further found that if the animal was first given breast cancer and then injected with estrogen, the hormone had a propensity to be taken up by some of the cancer cells. A protein inside the cancer cell was necessary to receive the incoming estrogen. This protein was named estrogen receptor (ER). However, in many cancer cells it was not present and consequently the estrogen was not taken up by those malignant cells.

By the early 1970's investigators had shown that some 60 to 70 percent of the human breast cancer cells contained estrogen receptor protein. This suggested that the cancer was estrogen dependent, and in the premenopausal patient if estrogen was denied the body by removing the ovaries, a remission of cancer was theoretically possible. As it turned out, however, only about half of these women were helped by removal of the ovaries. Further study revealed that it wasn't an all or nothing situation. Cancer cells had different levels of estrogen receptors. When the level was quantified, then one noted that if a patient's cancer cells had a very high level of ER, response to hormonal manipulation would be 65 percent. If the ER was absent or very low, the response was only 6 percent.

Building on these observations, it was soon discovered that progesterone receptors also occurred in breast cancer cells. Progesterone, another ovarian hormone, when placed in proximity to cancer cells, would enter those that contained a progesterone receptor. One could correlate the likelihood of hormone response to the presence of progesterone receptor. Patients that have both ER and progesterone receptor positive cancer cells have about an 80 percent favorable response to hormonal and chemotherapy treatment.[28]

Consequently, a check of the ER level and progesterone receptor level of cancer removed at surgery is a must, since only an average or high titer of ER level would pose a rational basis to prescribe removal of the ovaries. Should the pre-menopausal woman with metastatic breast cancer be ER positive of high titer, she would have a 65 percent chance of responding to ovariectomy by surgery or radiation.

The ER positive women who are fortunate enough to respond to the initial hormonal manipulation may find further control with chemotherapy and the anti-estrogen Tamoxifen (See Chapter 9).

The DNA Index: Desoxyribonucleic acid (DNA) found in the nucleus of every human cell is important in rendering a prognosis in breast cancer.[20] Cancer cells rapidly grow and multiply. During this rapid cell multiplication period, called the synthesis phase, DNA from the cell nucleus spills out and it can be measured such that the increase in DNA is proportional to the rapidity of cancer cell multiplication. Normal cells divide in an orderly manner with a predictable DNA production. This is a so-called diploid population of cells. By definition it is given an index of 1.0. Cancer cells divide so fast, we call them an aneuploid population of cells. The index may be anywhere between 1.0 and 2.0. The higher the index the more aggressive the cancer.

The S-Fraction: That proportion of cells undergoing rapid multiplication and growth during this synthesis phase is called the S-Fraction. The greater the S-Fraction, the greater proportion of malignant cancer cells are present that are aggressive and dangerous. At the same time of enhanced DNA production, a high S-Fraction reflects the proliferative capacity of a cancer, and thus its high growth rate and tendency to spread. The DNA Index and the S-Fraction are both used to determine the prognosis in a given case. These test results are used to prescribe or withhold treatments such as Tamoxifen and chemotherapy. However, for African-American women it has been demonstrated that the S-Fraction and DNA ploidy have no bearing on prognosis as is the case in white women. Hence, withholding of treatment should not be based on these tests for black women.[35]

Prostatic specific antigen (PSA) is generally used as a screening test for prostate cancer. It so happens that this same antigen is found in normal breast tissue and in breast cancers with a favorable prognosis.[25]

In all of these careful investigations to uncover the breast cancer perpetrator, the physician must be knowledgeable and persistent just like Holmes the detective. The investigation must be organized in a logical and straight-forward manner leading to the diagnosis. This can better be achieved successfully with the cooperation of the patient herself.

———

It is true, we cannot predict who will contract breast cancer. At the same time all of us must be aware of various premonitory conditions. In the next chapter you will have an opportunity to examine those risk factors as I attempt to examine the question: 'Who Gets Breast Cancer'?

CHAPTER FOUR

HE FICKLE FINGER OF FATE
Who Gets Breast Cancer?

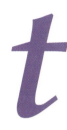he incidence of *lung* cancer among women is gaining with 46,000 new cases in 1985 and over 74,000 new cases found in 1995; and the rate is expected to continue to rise before decreasing as a result of the anti-smoking thrust sweeping the nation. Those numbers are impressive; but they are not even close to the epidemic of breast cancer.

In 1975, 70,000 new cases of breast cancer were discovered in the United States. In 1981, 109,000 cases were found. By 1985 119,000 new cases were added. Then in 1989 we saw 143,000 new breast cancer patients. In 1990 the figure rose to over 150,000 and in 1991 175,000 new cases were reported. The American Cancer Society estimated 182,000 new cases would be found in the United States in 1993.[38]

In 1996, the American Cancer Society projected 184,300 new cases and 44,300 deaths.[58] One out of every eight American women, without considering race, carry a lifetime risk for contracting breast cancer. There can be no doubt: Breast cancer is by far the number one cancer facing all women in the United States.

The National Cancer Institute reported that breast cancer in 1973 was diagnosed in 65.6 black women and 82.9 white women per hundred thousand population. However, before age 40, black women experience relatively more breast cancer than white women. By 1981 the overall number of black women with breast cancer had increased by 12 percent to 75 per hundred thousand while the incidence among whites had increased only 6 percent.[1] Other government studies emphasize the diminishing difference in the occurrence of breast cancer between black and white women.[2]

At the same time the mortality has always been higher in African-

American women. It appears that the mortality gap between the races is actually widening. In 1992 mortality among black women was 10 percent higher than whites.**42** In 1995 the American Cancer Society reported that mortality in blacks was 16 percent higher than whites.**49**

These figures point up the likelihood that black women are contracting breast cancer at a rate such that the relative number will soon surpass the occurrence among white women and the mortality gap will continue to widen. The National Cancer Institute revealed that between 1989 and 1993, breast cancer mortality for white women decreased by 6 percent but increased by 3 percent for black women.**59**

The problem of breast cancer is particularly acute among *young* black women when you consider the prevalence of cancer before the age of 40. An early study showed that from age 35 to 39 the incidence of breast cancer is 69.5 among blacks, compared to 59.0 for whites per hundred thousand population.**1** A more recent study revealed that before age 35 the incidence among black women is one and a half times the rate in white women.**41**

There is little wonder that women—rich and poor, black and white—are at least concerned if not downright alarmed.

I remember a young black woman timidly raising her hand during a question-answer period following one of my presentations. After she was recognized, she stood and in a small voice asked, "How will I know if I'm likely to get breast cancer, other than being a woman? I mean is there any thing that makes me more apt to get cancer than the next woman. You know what I mean? Is it just luck or something? You know what I mean?"

The young woman was asking, in her own way, 'What are the risk factors for getting breast cancer? What can we look for and prepare for, or is it just the fickle finger of fate?'

For most women there are no over-riding risk factors that we can identify. Researchers have shown that there are no known risk factors in 70 percent of breast cancer cases. On the other hand there are risk factors in 20 percent of younger women and in about 30 percent of older women.**38**

Let us review those markers that we know may increase your likelihood of acquiring breast cancer.

RISK FACTORS FOR BREAST CANCER

Advancing Age

In Europe and in the United States breast cancer rates are directly proportional to advancing age. American women, in general, at age 65 are more prone to cancer than those at age 40. There is a 30 fold increase in breast cancer risk from age 25 to 65. **3,4**

The Howard University experience reflects a different age distribution of breast cancer among black women. Cancer occurs at an earlier age. The rate at age 25 to 40 is similar to the breast cancer rate at 75 years and beyond.**43**

Heredity

It has long been recognized that some breast cancer patients, both black and white, are clustered in families such as sisters—mother and sister(s)—mother and daughter(s).**5**

Before the menopause these breast cancers with family ties are more often found than cancers that occur after the change of life. Hence, the pre-menopausal woman whose mother had breast cancer before her change of life will have a three fold increased chance of also developing breast cancer. A woman with a mother who had breast cancer after her menopause will have only a 1.2 increased risk of breast cancer. Investigators at the M.D Anderson Hospital in Houston examined the relatives of post-menopausal cancer patients who had cancer in both breasts. They found that close relatives had a four-fold increase in breast cancer. Close relatives of pre-menopausal women who had cancer in both breasts had a nine-fold increased risk of breast cancer.**5**

Without taking menopause into account, statistics show that a woman in the United States, with a sister or mother with breast cancer, carries a lifetime risk of one in five of contracting breast cancer. If the sister and mother both had breast cancer then the woman's lifetime risk of getting breast cancer increased to one chance in two. Her breast cancer would most likely strike before age 40 and would often be in both breasts.**6** As mentioned earlier, genetic factors seem to affect risk more often before menopause when ovarian estrogen plays a major role. Probably environmental factors take over the causative role in later life.**5**

Please read Chapter Five for a discussion of newly discovered genes that are directly related to breast cancer.

Female Sex vs Male Sex

It is true that females have an overwhelming number of breast cancers compared to males. Consequently, the female sex, per se, is a risk factor. The National Cancer Institute reported that in the five year period 1973 through 1977, the rates were 72 black females per hundred thousand compared to 1.4 black males per hundred thousand.**2** While breast cancer incidence has increased in women over the past 40 years, there has been no corresponding increase in male breast cancer. However, black men have a disproportionate higher mortality compared to white men.**2**

Testicular abnormalities such as undescended testicles, orchitis (infection in the testicles), or testicular injury, may predispose a man to breast cancer. Occupations in which the testicles are exposed to heat such as in steel mills and blast furnaces, seems to be associated with increased male breast cancer; and genetic influence similar to female breast cancer may also be operative.

Nevertheless, male breast cancer is so rare that many physicians complete their entire medical careers without seeing a single case. The concern is that a man may harbor a breast lump, suspecting some benign misfortune when a cancer is actually growing and spreading. As a result, studies reveal, most breast cancers in the male are large and have metastasized when finally diagnosed. The mortality is correspondingly high, simply because this rare male cancer was never suspected in its early stage.

Injury

Some women report a lump in the breast after a minor injury that draws their attention, leading them to carefully palpate the breast. If the lump they discover subsequently proves to be cancerous, the inference follows that the injury may have caused the cancer. As far as I am aware, there are no studies that demonstrate a causal link between injury and cancer of the breast. The injury caused by chapped and cracked nipples seen in the nursing breast and in non-pregnant women can cause infection; but, apparently, it does not lead to cancer. However, a bruise can lead to a lump of fat necrosis which may be indistinguishable from breast cancer even on mammogram and will thus require biopsy.

Parity

This refers to the number of children a woman has borne. Having a child at age 20 or younger decreases the chance of breast cancer significantly and having a child before age 30 also confers some protection. After the first child there is no further protection in having more children.[7] On the other hand, a first child born after age 35 triples the risk of breast cancer.[8] In the general population a woman who is nulliparous, that is, who has never carried a child to full term is at greater risk for breast cancer.[8] However, in the Howard University experience among black breast cancer patients there was no particular increased risk in women who had never had a child.[43]

Breast Feeding

Studies have failed to show a consistent relationship between breast

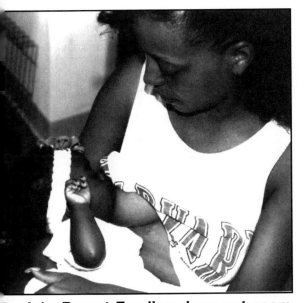

feeding or the lack of breast feeding and the subsequent development of breast cancer. One investigation from Japan (a low risk country) suggested there was some protection in prolonged breast feeding where lactation up to 5 to 10 years occurs frequently.[8] A review of the world-wide literature would indicate that prolonged nursing probably has little if any effect on the incidence of breast cancer. The Howard University study generally supports these conclusions. They found no relationship between breast feeding and breast cancer in black women.[47]

g. 4-1. **Breast Feeding does not seem have a bearing on the development of reast cancer. Nor does it protect against breast cancer.**

Radiation

There is no doubt that radiation can cause breast cancer.[9] Indeed radiation exposure can increase the incidence of cancer 2 to 3 times. That is why chest x-rays must be kept to a minimum and the dosage of mammography carefully controlled. A study reported in 1965 revealed that women who received multiple fluoroscopic examinations had a high incidence of breast cancer over a ten-year period.[10] It was also shown that the cancer developed on the side of the chest that received the radiation.

Other data examined Japanese women exposed to the radiation from the atomic blasts over Hiroshima and Nagasaki.[11] After observing this group for ten years, the investigators concluded that women exposed to 90 rads or more of radiation would develop breast cancer at a rate two to four times that of an otherwise comparable population.

Hodgkin's Disease treated with radiation under age 15 increases the risk of breast cancer. By age 24 to 29 radiation of Hodgkins's patient, breast cancer risk is 7 times that of the general population.[62]

Fibroadenoma

This is a common solitary benign tumor found in young women usually between the ages of 15 and 25. This tumor until recently was considered unrelated to breast cancer. However, in a report in 1994, investigators declared a link to subsequent invasive breast cancer if proliferative breast disease is also present. In such cases mammographic examination beginning at age 35 would be warranted.[71]

Proliferative Breast Disease

Sometimes called "benign breast disease," this group of conditions include sclerosing adenosis and hyperplasia (fibrocystic disease without atypia). If your biopsy reveals either one of these entities, it suggests only a slight increased risk of developing breast cancer. Regular breast self-examination, regular physical exams and mammography should be adequate follow-up.

Fibrocystic Dysplasia with Atypia

There seems to be a definite relationship between this type of fibrocystic dysplasia (cystic mastitis) and breast cancer. Although the mechanism remains unclear, several reports agree that women with fibrocystic dysplasia with atypia develop cancer four times as often as otherwise normal women.**12,13**

Breast cancer and fibrocystic dysplasia, it is believed, are induced by estrogen, the hormone produced by the ovary. The reason why some women respond to this hormone and develop benign fibrocystic dysplasia and others go on to malignant breast cancer is unknown. In some cases fibrocystic dysplasia forms so many dense nodules in the breasts it may be impossible to distinguish a cancer by palpation alone. Mammography may be useful although many times biopsy of a suspicious nodule is required for proper diagnosis.

ig. 4-2. Fibrocystic dyspla-ia. A biopsy will reveal if here is atypia which ncreases the risk of cancer.

Reports confirm, fibrocystic dysplasia and other benign breast diseases represent significant markers for possible development of cancer if there is atypia or cell abnormalities found in the biopsy specimen. Remember, even without atypia, there is a modest increased incidence of cancer developing.**40**

Lobular Carcinoma in Situ (LCIS)

This is one of the clearest markers of the possibility of cancer developing in a breast. In the past several years with the increased use of mammography this lesion is found more and more. It cannot be felt by simple palpation. It usually appears as a cluster of calcium grains on a routine mammogram. When LCIS is confirmed at biopsy, one can be sure that in 20 to 30 percent of cases a cancer will develop in either breast over a lifetime. This requires very careful mammograms yearly or more frequently. Some patients, particularly with a strong family history of breast cancer choose bilateral mastectomy rather than take the risk. I consider this to be a drastic option since the incidence increases only 1 percent per year for the first ten years.

Cancers associated with Breast Cancer

Cancer in one **breast** predisposes a woman to cancer in the opposite breast, and thus, presents a risk factor. Ten percent of breast cancer patients will develop cancer in the opposite breast, and depending on the cellular type, the rate may be higher. Indeed, it has been reported that a biopsy of the normal breast in the spot that cancer was found in the cancerous breast revealed hidden cancer in the normal breast in 20 percent of cases.[5]

There is a direct relation between cancer of the **uterus** and breast cancer. Apparently, estrogen or other unknown factors that lead to malignant degeneration of the uterine lining are also associated with breast malignancy. This combination occurs twice as often as noted in the general population. Hence, in every patient with proven cancer of the uterus, careful surveillance for breast cancer is mandatory and vice-versa.

Cancer of the **ovary** and breast cancer also arise together more often than expected by chance alone, but the association is more tenuous than the breast cancer-uterine cancer connection.

Ovarian cancer and uterine cancer are also found together for unknown reasons. A common stimulus is suspected since these cancer combinations, when they do occur, are found within a few years of one another.

Just as mysterious and fickle is the association of breast cancer and **colon** cancer. Some workers have shown that breast cancer follows the discovery of colon cancer more often than expected. So colon cancer is considered a risk factor. Populations at risk for colon malignancies, primarily Europeans and those ascribing to the diet of western cultures, consume a high fat content in their foods and this leads to a bacterial flora in the intestines which produces steroid compounds and estrogens which may be carcinogenic (able to cause cancer) for both colon and breast.

There is some association between breast cancer and **leukemia**. It has been noted that Hodgkins's disease in childhood can be associated with breast cancer by age 31.[44,45] There is some evidence that it is the radiation used to treat the Hodgkin's disease that may be the direct cause of later breast cancer.[52]

Finally, cancer of the **salivary glands** increases the likelihood of breast cancer by four in both black and white women.

Female Hormones Produced in the Body and Breast Cancer

We know that the hormone, estrogen, produced in the ovary is responsible for the female persona: the smooth hairless face, the rounded contoured physiognomy, the development of breast tissue, and menstruation. In Chapter Two it was pointed out that the onset of menstruation signals a sharply increased flow of estrogen from the developing ovaries; and we know that the longer a woman is exposed to estrogen the greater the chance of contracting breast cancer. Investigators have confirmed that females who begin menstruating early, perhaps at age nine or ten, and women who have a late menopause at age 55 instead of 45, will have an increased risk of cancer simply because they were exposed to estrogen a few years longer.

Conversely, women who have had their ovaries removed by surgery before the menopause have less breast cancer because of the shorter exposure time to estrogen. Males produce only minute amounts of estrogen, and develop breast cancer at a rate less than one percent of that found in the female. Men who have lost testicular function by injury or disease, or have undescended testicles are more likely candidates for breast cancer, as mentioned in a previous section. In experimental animals such as mice, hamsters and rabbits, breast cancer can be produced without fail by the injection of estrogen. All of these facts point to the central role of estrogen in producing human breast cancer.

Looking further, we find that there are actually three types of estrogen produced by the ovary: Estrone, Estradiol, and Estriol. This is important to understand since only the estrone and estradiol fractions are carcinogenic. Estrone and estradiol regularly produce breast cancer in the laboratory animal.

Estriol, however, not only fails to cause cancer, it can inhibit the estrone and estradiol estrogens.**14**

Ovaries of black Africans, Orientals and other non-whites produce mostly estriol. In Caucasians, the estrone and estradiol fractions are the predominant hormones. The high rates of breast cancer in whites compared to the rarity in black Africans and Orientals corresponds to the prevalence of estrone and estradiol in Caucasians and the predominance of estriol in non-whites. This finding was confirmed when comparing the estrogens of black Africans, whites and Indians in Zambia. Another study compared the estrogen types in Japanese women to those of a white population. The ovaries of white women produce these estradiol and estrone fractions more than any other race and they produce the vast majority of breast cancer.**15**

During pregnancy, the ovaries of all women, both black and white begin to elaborate large quantities of estriol, the safe estrogen. If pregnancy takes place before age 19, this surge of estriol will give a measure of protection against any breast cancer that would have occurred before age 45.

Incidentally, in male breast cancer there is elevated levels of estradiol, which is suspected of being a causal factor in male breast cancer.**56**

A study from Brazil in 1971 demonstrated that women whose first pregnancy was before age 20 had only one half the breast cancer risk as women whose first pregnancy was after age 25.**16**

Dr Henry M Lemon at the University of Nebraska has shown quite dramatically that estriol can prevent estrone and estradiol from causing breast cancer in animals.**14** Dr Lemon described the high incidence of estrone and estradiol in breast cancer patients and he wondered aloud if we shouldn't give estriol (the anti-cancer estrogen) to help prevent cancer in women who have low levels of this hormone.**17** Clearly this question can only be addressed through clinical trials.

You might ask, "If breast cancer is caused by female hormones, why does the cancer incidence continue to rise in older women after the ovaries stop producing hormones?"

No one has the complete answer, although there are credible theories. With the menopause or change of life, the estrogen level drops off as the ovaries begin to involute and atrophy. At that point the fickle finger beckons the adrenal and pituitary glands to take over and produce hormones that can be just as provocative in the development of breast cancer.

The adrenals, one small gland located above each kidney, manufactures a host of hormones, many of which are absolutely essential to life. They also produce some non-essential hormones including androstenidione and our old friend estrone, which, you will recall, is one of the cancer-causing estrogens.

Only 2 percent of the estrone is produced directly by the adrenals. Ninety eight percent is produced indirectly by way of the androstenidione.[18]

After the menopause, androstenidione, from the adrenal glands, has the capacity and does indeed produce estrone from the body's fat cells; and the more fat depots present the more estrone can be manufactured, and consequently, the greater potential for breast cancer.

It should be noted that androstenidione also induces the pituitary gland, located on the under surface of the brain, to secrete prolactin.

Prolactin, produced by the pituitary gland in the brain, is a hormone that is essential for the production of breast milk. It also promotes cancer in the presence of estrone. Some patients with breast cancer have high blood levels of prolactin. In fact close family members of some breast cancer patients have elevated prolactin levels. This may serve as a marker of relatives (mother, daughter, sister) that require special observation for cancer development.[18,19]

Hypophysectomy (surgical removal of the pituitary gland) has been an effective palliative treatment of metastatic breast cancer, probably due to the elimination of prolactin. Effective drugs that will bring consistent and sustained lowering of prolactin levels are being tested. Thus far, no drug that lowers prolactin level has proven to be satisfactory for breast cancer control.

Prescribed Hormones for Hot Flashes and Breast Cancer

For more than fifty years American women have been spared the nuisance and sometimes anguish of the menopause through the judicious use of hormones. These hormones, of course, are estrogens or estrogen-like medications. They have an excellent record of controlling the hot flashes, insomnia, perspiration, and anxiety that are sometimes a part of the change of life. In view of the carcinogenic consequences produced in the laboratory animal, a woman should be concerned about the propensity of these pills to cause human cancer.

A study from the Harvard School of Public Health is instructive. These investigators followed 1,891 menopausal women who were taking estrogens to alleviate hot flashes. These women were matched against the general population of the same age that were not taking the hormone. The groups were then observed over a fifteen-year period. For the first ten years there was no difference in the rate of breast cancer. After 12 years, it was noted that there was a 30 percent increased rate of breast cancer in those taking high doses of hormone for hot flashes.[20]

After 15 years of surveillance, women on high doses of estrogens showed twice the amount of breast cancer as the control group. Low-dose patients did not have a significant increment of breast cancer. This study also showed that breast cancer was higher in women that used estrogens three weeks out of the month rather than continuously. It has also been shown that hormone users that did develop breast cancer had a better prognosis with more being Estrogen Receptor Positive. See Chapter 3.

If fibrocystic dysplasia was present prior to using estrogens for menopausal symptoms, breast cancer occurred twice as often as the general population. If fibrocystic disease became evident following the use of these hormones, the fickle finger of cancer struck seven times more often than in the general population.[21]

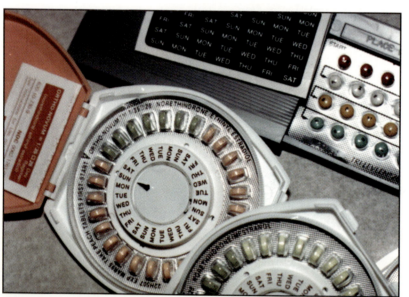

Fig. 4-3. Birth control pills may increase breast cancer risk in black women, particularly if there are other risk factors. There are conflicting reports when examining the general population.

Birth Control Pills and Breast Cancer

Medication produced for contraception generally contain an estradiol and/or an estrone-like hormone. Some also contain progesterone. The hormones in these medications are kept very low to avoid side effects. Women with known risk factors for breast cancer are cautioned to be extra vigilant. Package inserts clearly warn of the danger of birth control pills combined with such risk factors as fibrocystic dysplasia, prior history of breast cancer, or family history of breast cancer.

A study on the subject published in 1975 showed that women, black and white, who used oral contraception for two to four years increased their chances of contracting breast cancer two and a half times. Usage of less than two years or more than four years was not associated with increased risk. However, if benign fibrocystic disease was present and proven with biopsy then long-term use of birth control medication (six or more years) lead to an eleven-fold increase of breast cancer.[21]

An analysis by the Centers for Disease Control in 1982 suggested that oral contraceptives do not increase the risk of breast cancer. Their observations indicate that there is probably a beneficial effect in reducing the likelihood of contracting endometrial cancer (cancer of the womb).[22]

A more recent study reported from Howard University Hospital in 1993, revealed that among *black* women, use of birth control pills is clearly linked with increased risk of breast cancer.[47]

Much of the literature from Europe would link the use of oral contraceptives to breast cancer; and occasional articles in American journals also raise the association of breast cancer and birth control pills. Studies in 1996, examined a cohort of white women and found no association of breast cancer and birth control pills.[39-42]

All of this conflicting information gives you some idea of the differing experiences being reported, and the likelihood of confusion. My advice is to heed the package insert and avoid birth control pills if there are other risk factors present. If there are no other contraindications, then oral contraceptives represent a viable option for birth control. Nevertheless, there is enough data to warrant caution, particularly for black women.

Abortion and Breast Cancer

At the Fred Hutchinson Cancer Center in Seattle studies showed that women who had had an induced abortion were 50 percent more likely to develop breast cancer. Other investigators have not duplicated these results.[48] However, the Howard University Hospital studies of black women revealed a significant association of induced abortion and breast cancer in women older than 50 years of age. On the other hand spontaneous abortion or miscarriage seemed to have some protective effect from breast cancer.**47**

Pregnancy and Breast Cancer

It is often stated that pregnancy aggravates breast cancer and increases the likelihood of metastasis and death. This is not the case. Pregnancy does not stimulate the growth of breast cancer; and the prognosis is similar for pregnant and non-pregnant women.**63** The treatment is generally similar as in the non-pregnant stage--modified radical mastectomy or lumpectomy with axillary dissection. See Chapter 9. The only difference is that radiation and/or chemotherapy should be administered only after delivery of the baby. Termination of the pregnancy is only medically justified when there is a rapidly spreading cancer as in inflammatory breast cancer or if metastasis has already occurred and chemotherapy and radiation must be instituted immediately. Chemotherapy causes birth defects in a high rate of fetuses. Radiation is also detrimental to the fetus.

Subsequent pregnancy following treatment for breast cancer does not adversely affect the woman. Seventy percent of women, in child-bearing years, treated for breast cancer subsequently become pregnant on average 12 months after completing chemotherapy.**66** Sutton showed that 28 percent had recurrence of their cancer compared to 46 percent of women who did not become pregnant. It was also noted that mortality was less in women who became pregnant (12 percent vs 38 percent).**65**

Thyroid and Breast Cancer

The thyroid gland is an "H" shaped gland found in the neck. It produces thyroxine and other hormones that control the body metabolism. When the gland is overactive it sometimes enlarges forming a goiter and causing the heart to beat fast, the nerves to become tremulous, and weight loss in spite of a ravishing appetite. If the gland is underactive the body becomes sluggish and overweight. One becomes cold easily, the hair thins and face and hands become puffy.

In the post-menopausal years women are prone to have an underactive thyroid and are often placed on thyroid supplement medication. A report appearing in the Journal of the American Medical Association in

1976 analyzed 635 patients who were receiving thyroid medication and compared them with 4,870 women not on thyroid medication. These populations were followed for 15 years. Women on thyroid supplement had twice the rate of breast cancer as women not on thyroid medication. When the group on thyroid medication was broken down into women who had never bore a child and were on thyroid medication over 15 years, those women had a 33 percent excess risk of breast cancer. Women who had children had a 20 percent increased risk of breast cancer by virtue of using thyroid pills over 15 years. The conclusion of this study was that an underactive thyroid treated with thyroid extract for more than 15 years is a breast cancer risk factor.[23] Other studies also reveal a link between breast cancer and thyroid disease.[46]

Obesity, Diet and Breast Cancer

Following the menopause the incidence of breast cancer in the western culture continues to rise, while in Africa and the Orient the incidence, already low, drops even more to virtually zero in advanced years. The reason for this difference again may be the result of hormone influence stimulated by the western diet.

It has been shown that fat and obesity are directly related to breast cancer in later years.[24] If obesity is associated with hypertension and diabetes the incidence of breast cancer is further increased.[25]

The Body Mass Index (BMI) which considers height and weight gives some indication of breast cancer risk. The BMI is calculated by dividing body weight in Kilograms by the square of the height in meters times 100. Women with a BMI above 28 are at greater risk for breast cancer.[25]

> **BODY MASS INDEX**
> 1 pound equals .45 Kilogram and 1 inch equals .254 meter. Therefore if you weigh 200 pounds and are 63 inches tall your BMI would be: 200 X .45 divided by $(63 X .254)^2$ X100. That calculates to a BMI of 35. This is a BMI that carries an added risk for breast cancer developing.

The chemical dimethylbenzanthracene (DMBA) is used experimentally to induce breast cancer in mice. If the animal is placed on high fat rations, cancer is produced much faster and more predictably.[4]

Recent studies showed that a 30 year old woman who is ten pounds

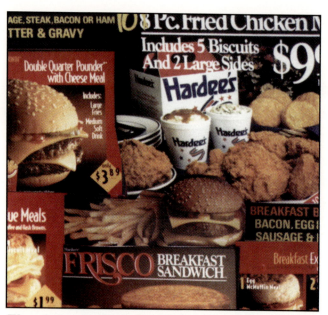

Fig. 4-4. A High Fat Diet is related to an increased likelihood of contracting breast cancer after age 50. Black women have the highest incidence of obesity in the United States.

overweight faces a 23 percent higher risk of developing breast cancer. If she is 20 pounds overweight the risk is 52 percent higher.**57**

This may help explain in part why black women are showing an accelerated incidence of breast cancer. African-American women have the greatest incidence of obesity in this country—more than black or white males and more than white women.

Earlier I mentioned that African black women rarely had breast cancer. The incidence is one tenth that of black women in the United States.**60** However, it has been demonstrated in South Africa that when the rural black woman moved to the city and assumed the western style high fat diet, the breast cancer rate began to increase sharply over a few years. Another study indicated that if one transplants the Japanese woman from her homeland to Hawaii with its western diet, one discovers the same inclination to increase the breast cancer rate in older women.**26** The rural African and Oriental diets average 40 grams of fat per day, while the westernized diet averages 140 to 180 grams of fat daily. In the state of Utah, where the low fat Mormon diet prevails in many sections, breast cancer in white women is lower than the national average.**27**

The Women's Health Initiative, a study being conducted by the National Institutes of Health, to be completed by 2005 will answer the question: "If a middle-age woman goes on a low fat diet, will the morbidity and mortality of breast cancer be altered?"

There is a growing belief that diet factors other than low fat are important in prevention and treatment of cancer. For example, it was discovered that women with breast cancer have lower tissue levels of Vitamins C and E.**67** Researchers found that women with terminal breast cancer had life extended 5 to 15 years when they took large doses of anti-oxidants such as Vitamin E and Vitamin C on a regular basis.**68**

Selenium is an essential mineral and has recognized cancer preventive qualities. Low levels of selenium are associated with breast cancer and other cancers. It has been shown in animal studies that Selenium can prevent breast cancer.**69**

Calcium has been shown in a recent Italian study to be important in breast cancer prevention.**70**

Finally, there is some evidence that Vitamin D and the B-complex vitamins and trace elements of copper and zinc may help stave off breast cancer. There is even evidence that soybean and cabbage may have poorly understood properties that fight cancer.

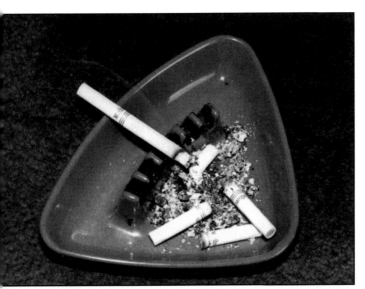

g. 4-5. Smoking and Breast Cancer may be ated in heavy smokers over a 30 year period of ne.

Smoking and Breast Cancer

Most medical studies refute the association of breast cancer and cigarette smoking; although a few reports suggest otherwise. One group examined the question on two occasions. The first study showed that smoking was associated with breast cancer and the second study found no correlation whatsoever.**28** A report in 1995 suggested that women who smoked for more than 30 years were 15 percent more likely to develop breast cancer compared to non-smokers. It was also shown that the average age of developing cancer was 59 years of age compared to 67 years in non-smokers.**55**

In November 1996, the media reported that a new study purported to relate smoking and breast cancer. Careful reading of the report revealed that women who are slow acetylators tend to metabolize carcinogens slower and allow cancer causing agents to damage the body for longer periods before metabolic elimination. So-called slow acetylators have a genetic basis that causes a slow liver metabolism of various medications, waste products and carcinogenic material in certain food additives and cancer-causing agents in tobacco smoke. There is a four-fold increase in breast cancer among post-menopausal smokers who are slow acetylators. This condition (slow acetylator) pertains to 40 percent of white women, but occurs less often in black women. 61

Alcohol Consumption and Breast Cancer

A recent study showed that even half a drink of alcohol per day increased the risk of breast cancer. The intensity of consumption was most important while the duration was of less importance. Reducing alcohol intake may reduce the risk of breast cancer.72

Environment/Occupation and Breast Cancer

The association of occupation and the environment and breast cancer has no proven causal link, but associations continue to stimulate interest and suggest the need for further scientific evaluation.

For example, there is an increased association among teachers and nurses with breast cancer. Also receptionists, cosmetologists, and textile workers.50

A recent study found that women exposed to high doses of electro-magnetic fields (EMF), such as main frame computers and power lines had a 40 percent excess risk of breast cancer. Average low levels of EMF such as found in home appliances were of no consequence. For years investigators have tried to show an association with exposure to overhead high voltage power lines and breast cancer. Heretofore the results have been either ambiguous or have shown a weak association. In this present study, after factoring in all known risk factors, the investigators found an 84 percent increase in the incidence of breast cancer in young women highly exposed to EMF. In post menopausal women the increased risk was 32 percent. The only problem with the study was that the number of women studied was small which increases is the possibility that the association was due to chance.**53**

Interesting studies relating the pesticide DDT and breast cancer have been reported. Although DDT was banned in 1972, it is still present in our bodies, stored in our fat cells. Black, white and Asian women were compared for the presence of DDT and the chance of breast cancer. For the white and Asian women there was no statistical correlation. However, for black women there was indeed a statistical correlation; and the more DDT present the more breast cancer. Black and Asian women were also found to have a significantly higher level of poly-chlorinated biphenyls (PCB). PCB, along with 200 other chemicals and pesticides are being scrutinized for a breast cancer association. The most suspicious associations thus far include styrene, methylene chloride, carbon tetrachloride (used in dry cleaning), formaldehyde, acid mists and metal oxides.**51**

Since 1995 the National Cancer Institute, in conjunction with the National Institute of Environmental Health Sciences, has funded six environmental studies that include PCB and DDT. The bulk of this effort is centered in the Northeast and mid-Atlantic States where breast cancer is above the national average. The NCI Long Island Breast Cancer Project is one of the six projects currently in progress.

Racial Genetics and Breast Cancer

As mentioned earlier black African women rarely contract breast cancer; but in the United States breast cancer is occurring in epidemic proportions among black women. You might wonder, 'Why this difference? If cancer of the breast is so rare among our black African sisters, why is it so prevalent in American black women? Are we not essentially the same people, or are we so different? Or is it simply the fickle finger of fate?'

The American Negro, if you will, is a hybrid group in the United States that began shortly after the first slaves were brought to America around 1619. The genetic pool of the pure strain black African was blended with the Indian or native American, the Hispanic, and most of all the European white slave master. The Negro hybrid race flourished with continual addition of Caucasian genes during the antebellum era and even unto this day we witness a continued blending of the races, and an admixture of the genetic pool.

For a long time we were unable to accurately measure the amount of Caucasian genetic mixture in a population of black Americans. Then someone noted that the whites had more blood type A than blacks. With this marker one could roughly estimate the degree of Caucasian mixture in a large population of blacks. This was only a very crude supposition since various groups of pure strain Africans had differing amounts of type A blood. Then, in 1969 there was a breakthrough of sorts. Dr T. Edward Reed, a Canadian geneticist persuasively demonstrated the usefulness of the Caucasian gene Fa of the Duffy blood group. This so-called Duffy gene is prevalent in all Caucasians and virtually absent in pure strain black Africans.[29]

It so happens that the gene is exclusively a Caucasian phenomena and if the Duffy gene is found in a population of hybrid Negroes, one could accurately estimate the percentage of Caucasian admixture in that population.

Dr. Reed next examined black people in the northern United States for the presence of the Duffy gene and compared this with the presence of the Duffy gene in a population of southern blacks. He showed that liver cirrhosis due to alcohol abuse was found in whites and only in blacks with the Duffy gene. He predicted that other diseases in Negroes would probably be found in addition to liver cirrhosis that would be tied to the Caucasian admixture.

The following year Dr. Nicholas Petrakis, at the University of California Medical School in San Francisco used Reed's conclusions to examine the incidence of breast cancer in black American women.[30] First ,he observed that black Ugandans and Nigerians had virtually no trace of the Duffy gene and a breast cancer rate of 9.5 per hundred thousand—an extremely low rate. Then he measured the Duffy gene frequency in American whites and found it to be present in all cases. The breast cancer incidence in white American women in that particular year was 69 per hundred thousand, one of the highest rates in the world. Finally, Dr Petrakis measured the Duffy gene frequency in three populations of black women in Detroit, Atlanta, and Oakland, California. He also measured the frequency of breast cancer in these populations. His findings which were statistically significant showed that the northern black women had a greater admixture of the Caucasian Duffy gene and a proportionately greater incidence of breast cancer which corroborated Reed's findings.

In other words he discovered that black populations with a greater presence of the Duffy gene had more breast cancer, proportional to the extent of the white genetic admixture.

Socio-economic Status and Breast Cancer—Risk or Fate?

Socio-economic status (SES) is a conglomeration of such variables as median family income, years of formal education, number of family dependents, and other related measurements. Statisticians have attempted with some success to relate an increased chance for breast cancer with a higher SES. They have gone to some length with statistical machinations to show that women who have a college education and high income have more breast cancer than poor blacks. This notion will soon have to be modified as the incidence of breast cancer in blacks continues to soar and will probably exceed the frequency in the white community. As already mentioned, the incidence is already much higher in black women under age 40, in spite of a lower SES.

Epidemiologists and their statistician colleagues have also demonstrated that survival after cancer diagnosis favors those of the higher SES and, of course, these are predominantly white women. I find difficulty with the notion that education or money actually affects the number of cases of breast cancer.

I also take issue with the idea that simply by the accident of being black condemns one to a poor prognosis. The question is, "Is survival actually due to SES or is SES simply a marker for some other causative factor?" On closer scrutiny one finds that women with a high SES, who are more often Caucasian, are likely to be nulliparous (never born a child), or they had a first child at an older age. They probably use hormones for one reason or another, and exist on a high fat diet. There is also the predominant estrogen type produced that is carcinogenic. These are additive possible risk factors for breast cancer. The SES is simply a marker.

As for the poor prognosis for black women, McWhorter and his associates reporting in the American Journal of Public Health in 1987 studied 36,905 breast cancer cases.[35] They found that black women with breast cancer received less aggressive treatment. They were most likely to either have no surgery or certainly no cancer-directed treatment. However, this difference was more related to poverty than race. I say it can be related to either since poverty and racism so often exist together. For example, Farrow reported in 1992 that African-American women were less likely to receive radiation therapy after surgery although it is known that post-op radiation treatment favorably affects recurrence.[71]

A report from the American Cancer Society in 1986 concluded that socio-economic status (SES) rather than race determined survival after a cancer diagnosis.[31] If that's the case, then blacks and whites who contract breast cancer and share a similar high socio-economic status should like-wise share a similar favorable prognosis. They do not! If you are black, rich, and educated, your prognosis will not be nearly as favorable as your white counterpart.[32,33]

On the other hand, when looking at other cancers in which blacks have a poor prognosis such as bladder, prostate, and uterus, race, undeni-ably, remains the predominant factor. In a study by Mayer in 1989, it was shown that black patients regardless of SES were more likely to go untreat-ed following a diagnosis of bladder and other cancers with a predictably grave outcome.[36]

An earlier paper by Wynder and his associates in studying only white women showed there was no difference in breast cancer incidence or survival based on SES. In other words poor whites and rich whites con-tracted breast cancer at the same rate and fared equally after treatment.[34]

An article in the Journal of the National Cancer Institute in 1992 revealed that black women, without considering SES, were more likely to have advanced breast cancer when first diagnosed, with a corresponding high mortality.[37]

Many investigators agree that if there is a socio-economic basis for the dismal outlook for black women, it is the poverty component, borne of racism, that appears to be the key.

We know that the entry into the medical market-place for poor black families is more cumbersome and discouraging. Transportation may be a problem. The hours spent in overflowing waiting rooms, beset by cold, indifferent clerks and receptionists, can be a harrowing experience as small children and chores go unattended. With the tide of Health Maintenance Organizations (HMO's) engulfing the nation, health care chaos, I predict, will become a calamity.

Why the economically disadvantaged should be doomed to a higher mortality has never been answered or squarely confronted. Even when you match the disadvantaged, at whatever stage of disease you find them, against the socio-economically advantaged at a comparable stage of disease, and add the race variable, the poor regularly exhibit a higher mortality.

Why are we losing so many women—poor and black or rich and black for that matter—to breast cancer? I suspect, and the data suggests, that the overall medical care and attention offered this group is less than optimum—to say the least.

In a society where black infant mortality is almost twice that of white babies in 1998, and statistics all along the line bear out the racial dichotomy, I would venture that pervasive racism seeping through the medical establishment, frustrates even fundamental efforts of health care delivery to people of color.

It is the crowded inner-city clinics catering to the poor and the black where one finds the most complications and the highest mortality figures in breast cancer and other diseases. In the medical arena as elsewhere in our society, the cannon fodder remains the same. In the foreseeable future, the fickle finger will continue to point to the combination 'black and poor' as a special risk category in the breast cancer dilemma.

————

Not only does race and poverty present a special risk factor, but in more than 10 percent of breast cancers, heredity must be considered. In the coming years, I suspect that genetics will be found to be disproportionately of greater significance in black women. These suspicions will be discussed in the next chapter when we discover that breast cancer can be a family affair.

Therefore, I say unto you, Be not anxious for your life, what ye shall eat, or what ye shall drink; nor yet for your body, what ye shall put on. Is not life more than food and the body than raiment...seek ye first the kingdom of God and his righteousness, and all these things shall be added unto you. Be...not anxious about tomorrow; for tomorrow will be anxious for the things of itself. .....

Matthew 6: 25,31..34

CHAPTER FIVE

WHEN BREAST CANCER IS ALL IN THE FAMILY
Genetics and Breast Cancer

 believe that the genes you are born with play a greater role in the incidence of breast cancer among African American women than in the general population. This has not been specifically proven at this time, but available evidence points towards that conclusion. For one thing breast cancer tends to occur at an earlier age in black women, which is also characteristic of familial breast cancer. It is also an accepted fact that breast cancer is more aggressive, and metastasizes early on in black women. This is equally characteristic of hereditary breast cancer.

It is widely held that breast cancer is inherited in approximately 9 percent of cases.1 However in the Howard University Study 12.2 percent of black women reported a family history of breast cancer. 2 A study of black women at Harlem Hospital showed a 14 percent family history of breast cancer.11

A group at the University of Pennsylvania Fox Chase Cancer Clinic reported on early breast cancer in black and white women. They noted that Ductal Carcinoma in Situ (DCIS) is present in 12 percent of all cancers, almost always before the age of 40. This is a cancer that is discovered before it has begun to invade the surrounding breast tissue. They believe DCIS is influenced by genetics and that invasion is triggered by estrogen or other factors. These investigators point out that black women have a 1.84 increased risk of DCIS (almost twice the risk) over their white counter parts. This means an increased genetic influence in African-American women.14

Obviously detailed pedigree histories need to be obtained among all women with breast cancer and any racial differences investigated and documented.

In 1865 hereditary breast cancer was first described by the noted French physician Paul Broca. He observed that his wife had contracted breast cancer along with several women of her family going back four generations. But it wasn't until 1965, one hundred years later, that investigators began to systematically collect information about the family members of breast cancer patients and re-discovered a predilection to contract breast cancer based on heredity.

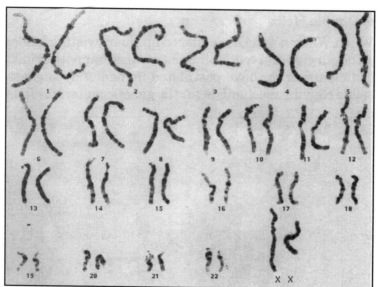

Fig. 5-1. Female chromosomes carry the genetic codes for breast cancer and many other diseases. Mapping of the entire gene pool (genome) is now feasible with the computer. The genetic basis of breast cancer is a fertile field for the next generation of scientists.

In September 1994, Dr Mark Skolnick at the University of Utah isolated a gene, later named BRCA1. That gene markedly increased the tendency to develop breast cancer. Shortly thereafter a second gene BRCA2 was discovered and linked to hereditary breast and ovarian cancers.

In addition to gene linkage there can be a family history without any culpable gene thus far discovered. From 5 to 20 percent of breast cancer patients found today, have either a strong family history, or identifiable genes (BRCA1 or BRCA2).

A woman who has two first degree relatives i.e. mother or sister, with breast cancer, will develop breast cancer three times as often as the general population. A specific gene will not be found in this group of women, but it is expected that more provocative genes will eventually be discovered. Such a family history puts these women at moderate risk. A strong family history places a woman at no more than 30 percent of excess risk of developing breast cancer in her life-time.

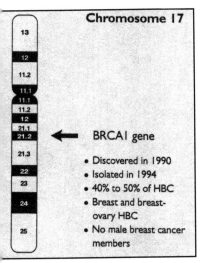

Chromosome 17

BRCA1 gene

- Discovered in 1990
- Isolated in 1994
- 40% to 50% of HBC
- Breast and breast-ovary HBC
- No male breast cancer members

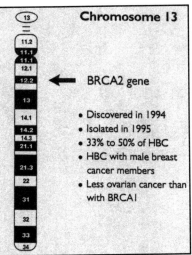

Chromosome 13

BRCA2 gene

- Discovered in 1994
- Isolated in 1995
- 33% to 50% of HBC
- HBC with male breast cancer members
- Less ovarian cancer than with BRCA1

Figs. 5-2 / 5-3.
Breast Cancer genes have been discovered on chromosomes 17 and 13. In the coming years many more genes will be discovered.

Other women, not only have family members with breast cancer, but they indeed share similar genes (BRCA1 or BRCA2) with those relatives, that places these women at high risk to develop breast cancer. While a test for the BRCA2 gene is not available yet, the BRCA1 gene can be detected by a simple blood test. Carriers of either gene (BRCA1 or BRCA2) have an 87 percent life time risk of developing breast cancer.

If a clinician strongly suspects a genetic basis in a family, a blood sample can be sent to a research laboratory to find out if a female member of that family carries the gene. Bear in mind that the cost is excessive and insurance coverage tenuous.

By reviewing the family histories of a woman and identifying the occurrence of breast, colon, and ovarian cancers in female and male relatives, one can assign a percentage to the likelihood of that asymptomatic female member acquiring breast cancer in her lifetime. In this way, women can be identified for special follow-up and surveillance before cancer is manifest. For those women with a positive family history, mammography should start at age 20 and continued on a yearly basis.

A clearly identifiable genetic basis for breast cancer is usually found when four or more close relatives had breast, colon or ovarian cancer, and the cancers develop before age 45, with a large proportion occurring between ages 25 and 35. Claus estimates that 36 percent of breast cancer contracted between ages 20-29 have a clear genetic basis. Others state that 50 percent of breast cancers under age 30 are hereditary.[3] These cancers are highly aggressive, and tend to grow rapidly and metastasize early. Black women, below age 35 contract breast cancer one and a half times the rate of white women. Therefore black women may have a greater hereditary predilection to breast cancer. The tumor size doubles in 157 days when the patient happens to be between the ages of 50 and 70. Over age 70 cancer grows more slowly and the doubling time is 188 days. By contrast cancer in women under age 50 are more aggressive. The doubling time is only 88 days, and even less in young women under age 35.

Risk assessment based on family history has been neglected until very recently with the discovery of genetic clues.4 The Claus Tables have been developed to assess an individual's chance of developing breast cancer. There are flaws in the procedure, but it does serve as a rather crude tool for estimating moderate risk.5

The Gail model, on the other hand, is used to estimate the chance of breast cancer in high risk women with a family history of breast, colon, or ovarian cancers. These patients in all likelihood have identifiable genes. Software based on the Gail model is available to graphically depict probability of breast cancer. As with the Claus tables, there are flaws and drawbacks. Two of the glaring problems with the Gail model is that it can only be applied to women receiving annual mammograms, and it is based on studies of white women, with black women specifically excluded.6

Nevertheless, the Gail model is being used to screen patients into the NSABP Breast Cancer Chemoprevention Trial. This is a study begun in 1992, designed to run five and ten years, to see if Tamoxifen can prevent or forestall the development of breast cancer in women at high risk. Black women are being recruited into this study based on criteria derived from data that excluded black women.

It is claimed that various adjustments have been made in the Gail model to allow the study of black women in the Tamoxifen trial.13 It is essential that black women be recruited for these Tamoxifen trials since the mortality among black women, in the past 20 years, has increased by over 5 percent more than whites. In post-menopausal black women the mortality rate has increased 22 percent more than in post-menopausal white women.7

Breast cancer risk assessment is an emerging service that includes determination of risk, recommendations for surveillance, counseling for at-risk individuals, and education regarding health promotion behavior.

Risk assessment centers are designed to: 1. Assess a woman's preconceived notions about cancer. 2. Discuss risk perceptions. 3. Construct a detailed pedigree. 4. Assess lifetime risk of breast cancer based on tables (Claus) and chance of gene BRCA1 and BRCA2 inheritance. 5. Begin surveillance 6. Identify families for genetic testing. 7. Provide psychological counseling.8

With this new capacity to determine if you carry a mutated gene that would indicate some certainty of developing breast cancer, many women are asking their doctors to find out if they carry the gene. After all, they reason, the patient has "a right to know".

INDICATIONS TO ADVOCATE TESTING

1. If a woman's mother was diagnosed with breast or ovarian cancer before age 50.

2. Any woman with at least three close relatives with breast or ovarian cancer

3. A woman with breast cancer under age 30 should be tested. If positive then close relatives should also be tested.

4. A woman of Ashkenazi Jewish heritage, with any female relative under age 40 with breast cancer, should be tested.

On the other hand some believe that genetic testing should not be done outside of a research protocol. They reason that we are still debating what the correct response to such information should be. Does one advocate bilateral mastectomy? Removal of the ovaries? Increased surveillance, or what? They also state that insurance companies may suddenly find a pretense to halt or modify medical coverage. Job security may be jeopardized. And what about the anxiety generated among other members of the family that will need to be tested? If a man or woman is found to have the mutated gene (BRCA1 or BRCA2) there is a 50 percent chance of passing it to an offspring.

Thus far there is no agency to monitor the accuracy of the testing procedure in private facilities. If the gene is found in a particular person, we do not know when breast cancer will arise. Even the estimate of cancer arising in a particular individual at all is imprecise. Thus there is no consensus of available treatment to recommend if the gene is found to be present.

Nevertheless, proponents for testing of anyone who desires the test, make a strong argument. First, the American Society for Clinical Oncology, a premiere organization of cancer specialists has gone on record favoring free access to testing. They point out that the 185delAG mutation of BRCA1 found in Ashkenazi Jewish women is extremely penetrant, and if found would demand that all female relatives be tested, since the risk for family members that carry the gene have an 85 percent lifetime risk of breast cancer and a 60 percent risk of ovarian cancer. Proponents for access to testing believe that women will be able to choose available options based on information. Some may opt for careful monitoring using the new imaging techniques now available as noted in Chapter 3. Others may choose radical surgery. Insurance and job discrimination, if they occur, should be challenged in the courts and on the political front.

In my opinion, there is no question that women should have access to this testing; and counseling must be available to interpret the findings and assist in choosing intelligent options. If women must depend on qualifying for a study protocol before being tested, it may be that whatever the researchers are studying at a particular time would disqualify a cohort of women who did not meet the criteria of the protocol, thus excluding a whole segment from knowing if they indeed have a strong genetic predisposition to breast cancer.

Experience teaches us that black women are generally the last to be included in any study protocol, especially screening and preventive trials. It stands to reason that black women would be at high risk of being deprived of genetic testing if limited to some research study. Most women, I suspect, will forego testing outside of a study protocol because of the high cost. One test may cost several thousand dollars and may not be covered by insurance.

The National Breast Cancer Coalition (NBCC) has declared that any woman who submits to genetic testing must agree to be part of a research protocol. Fran Visco, the president of NBCC states that the research protocol should be designed to answer such questions as, "What do we do with women who test positive? What kind of counseling do they need? How do we protect them from discrimination? Are there any prevention strategies?"[12]

Besides the hereditary breast cancer genes, there are other genes that may increase the chance of breast cancer indirectly. They are called suppressor genes, oncogenes, and proto-oncogenes.

The p53 is a harmless suppressor gene that suppresses breast cancer development. That's its job. But if p53 is damaged or altered it becomes dangerous and can no longer suppress or prevent breast cancer. This is particularly serious for black women. An alteration in the p53 gene does not affect prognosis in white women with breast cancer to the extent found in black women. For black women with an altered or mutated p53 gene, there is a five-fold increase in breast cancer deaths.[9] Thus it is important that the p53 marker be checked to help determine prognosis and treatment options in black women.

The c-erbB-2 is another gene of great interest. When present it may directly or indirectly lead to breast cancer. Its presence has not been consistently correlated with breast cancer prognosis, although one study showed that the higher expression of c-erbB-2 the better the patient responds to chemotherapy. Nevertheless firm conclusions regarding the meaning and usefulness of this gene in the diagnosis and treatment of early and late breast cancer have not been settled.[10]

While these new discoveries are fascinating and undoubtedly will augment our pursuit of the breast cancer villain, we must continue to press for mammography screening and urge breast self-examination.

———

As we shall see in Chapter 6, black women have consistently failed, for a variety of reasons, to take advantage of cancer screening opportunities; and this will require a special ongoing educational effort on the part of all of us.

Breast cancer screening should be an integral part of every health department in every community. If immunizations for measles and mumps can be provided mammography should also be available. If the health department can provide free Pap smears to detect early cervical cancer, then why not be as diligent in uncovering early breast cancer that kills three times as many black women before the age of thirty as cervical cancer.

Until The Public Health Department addresses this issue, African Americans blessed with abundant wealth must be offered the opportunity to participate in funding screening programs. Too many women are dying of breast cancer, unable to afford a screening mammogram.

Let us not forget "...for whomsoever much is given of him shall much be required..." (Luke 12:48)

CHAPTER SIX

NEEDLE IN THE HAYSTACK
Finding Breast Cancer

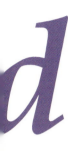iscovering breast cancer in the general population is like finding a needle in a haystack. For the private sector it would seem impractical, if not impossible, to screen the entire country on a regular basis. This is clearly a public health issue, since it must be continuous and ongoing. Presently there is inadequate government funding for screening mammography and only mediocre commitment.

Early attempts by the private sector to screen women for breast cancer on a large scale have been recorded. It began in the 1950's when x-ray mammography was not part of the screening process, only breast palpation and observation were done.[1] Investigators showed that breast cancer could be discovered in an early stage. Whether or not this increased the cure rate or just prolonged survival could not be said with certainty since there was no control group for comparison. To justify the time and public expense of large scale screening, it was imperative to prove that breast cancer mortality could be significantly reduced by comparing the results to a control group.

The first time such a control group was used for comparison was the Breast Cancer Screening Project of the Health Insurance Plan of Greater New York. This study commonly called the HIP project was begun in December 1963.[2] A population of women numbering 62,000, ages 40 to 64, was gleaned from the insurance registry of the State of New York and divided into two equal groups. These groups were closely matched with regards to age, marital status, number of children, benign breast disease, religion, and even education. No mention of race was made.

One group was screened for breast cancer in a periodic systematic manner, and the control group received only their customary medical attention. The screened group was examined yearly for cancer using x-ray mammography or physical examination. The enrollees were also instructed in breast self-examination. In 1972 after nine years of screening, the HIP project reported 30 percent less mortality from breast cancer in the screened group, when compared to the control group. Of the cancers found in the screened group, 33 percent were discovered only by mammography and 45 percent found by palpation alone. If the population was divided according to age groups, only 19 percent of cases in the 40-49 age category could be found by mammography alone. In the 50-59 age group, mammography alone was successful in 42 percent of cases. This finding was explained on the basis of the greater density of breast tissue in the younger women and the shortcomings of the x-ray equipment used in the 1963-1972 period. In the following decades using selenium plates and better equipment the mammogram yield would dramatically improve.

After the HIP project findings, the medical profession began to seriously speculate that finding the needle in the haystack was feasible, and clinicians around the country geared up for a massive screening to find hidden breast cancer. Nevertheless there were many hindrances. For one thing getting asymptomatic women, particularly black women, to come in for an examination and return periodically required much effort in solicitation and follow-up. There was no existing list of women from which to draw as in the HIP study. Another problem was cost effectiveness. The sheer number of medical personnel and support services to conduct the exams, compile the data, and analyze the statistics could prove to be a formidable task. Would it be economically feasible to find the needle in the haystack working through the private sector?

A screening project was set up by the Guttman Institute in New York in 1968 headed by Dr. Philip Strax.[3] Dr Strax designed his project to answer questions concerning feasibility of operation and cost effectiveness. The project was prepared to screen 50,000 women per year with an additional 15,000 screened through mobile units and out-reach programs. Not only were they supported by charitable gifts; but the American Cancer Society, New York Division, and the National Cancer Institute lent their combined assistance.

Using a new generation of mammographic machines and films, Dr

Strax and his associates were impressed with the capacity of mammography and physical examination to uncover cancers independently. When using these two modalities together, 95 percent of cancers were found on the initial screening. They also noted that women re-screened after only a year interval would show a cancer not previously picked up. It was estimated that 5 to 10 percent of unsuspected breast cancers were missed. However, those cancers missed would be discovered within a year by re-examination or by the patient herself discovering the suspicious lesion in the interim.

Dr Strax found that the requirements of an adequate screening project could be enormous. Some of the financial burden, however, could be curtailed by replacing doctors and nurses with health aides. These aides, some taken from the community served, were trained to carry out the entire project under proper supervision. The new mammography machines were simple in their design and required only a few weeks to master. A technician, it was learned, could be fully trained in about 4 weeks to begin breast inspection and palpation. It was shown that a technician, working with hundreds of mammograms, learned to spot the abnormal films quite handily. Out of a hundred films they would call ten abnormal. Almost always if a cancer was present in the hundred films, it would be in the ten chosen for further scrutiny. A cadre of vocational nurses and nurses aides were ideal for this purpose. This saved the trained physician-radiologist valuable time, and it was obviously cost-effective for the project. After five years, 1968-73, the cost was calculated to be approximately twenty dollars per patient.

Dr Strax and others began to realize that if the purpose of mass screening is to lower the death rate of breast cancer patients, then this must clearly be a public health issue that should be supported by public health tax dollars. As you can imagine, the public trough was crowded with many other worthy health causes—each vying for a preferential pecking order. Multiple sclerosis, The Heart Fund, Hypertension Screening, Maternal and Child Welfare, Drug Abuse—all depended, in large measure, on public funding.

Whenever a new program is evaluated for financial assistance the cost/benefit ratio is carefully examined before allocating scarce tax dollars.

There always seems to be ardent supporters of one cause or another.

Voluntary groups, in 1968, such as the Guttman Institute found little financial support from the government. Consequently, Dr Strax and the Guttman Institute pooled their resources with American Cancer Society volunteers to set up a screening program and advertised through the media (radio and print) that breast screening was available. Only 5.3 percent of those responding to the call for free breast screening were black women, numbering 14,864. Of that number, only 43.1 percent completed the five year screening, compared to 53 percent of the white women. In fact, after the first two annual exams, 32.6 percent of the black women had dropped out of the program, compared to 23.9 percent of the white group.

Even with this poor attendance breast cancer was found in 5.9 percent of the black women and 5.4 percent of the whites. Similar cancer detection rates between the races continued over the five-year period in spite of the fact that so many black women didn't bother to come back each year. We can only speculate on how many black women with breast cancer were missed because they did not return for follow-up. As it turned out, 80 percent of the breast cancers that were detected during the five-year period were very early and probably curable. This is twice the percent of black women who turn up at clinics and medical offices, in the general population, with early breast cancer.4

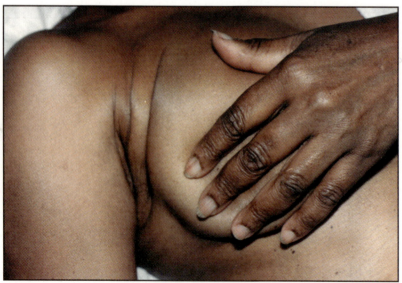

Fig. 6-1. Breast Self Examination (BSE) should be taught by your health provider. BSE should should be done on a monthly basis beginning at age 20.

The largest screening program for breast cancer to date was first reported in 1988. It was called the **Breast Cancer Detection Demonstration Project (BCDDP).5** In 1997 a twenty-year follow-up

A Needle in the Haystack

report was made. Between 1973 and 1980, 283,222 women, ages 35 to 74, were screened and 4,275 breast cancers were found. They were followed for up to twenty years.**14** Initially, the study was conducted under the auspices of The National Cancer Institute and The American Cancer Society. They joined forces and funded 29 centers throughout the country that began to screen women for breast cancer. One third of cancers found were fifty years of age or younger. Unfortunately, women under age forty were excluded in most of the calculations and the racial breakdown was

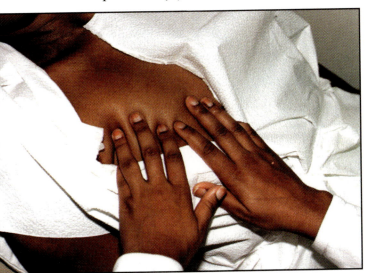

g. 6-2. Professional Examination every year and y time you discover a mass.Insist on a mammo- am regardless of age if you even "think" a lump present.

de-emphasized other than stating that statistics indicate that black women did not fare as well as their white enrollees.**15** Almost 42 percent of the cancers uncovered were found by mammography alone while physical examination alone found 8.7 percent.

In the HIP project of the 1960's, mammography alone detected about 33 percent of the cancers and 45 percent were detected by physical examination alone.**6** This difference is a result of the strides made in mammography which is now considered the major tool in finding very early unsuspected breast cancers.

The Guttman study was a noble endeavor. However, it only scratched the surface. With the resources now at our disposal it is simply not feasible for private clinics to screen such a huge target population on a regular basis. The haystack is too great, the needle too small, and the searchers too few. Nevertheless with the available screening technology now available, 30 percent more women could be saved even without further research; the needle could be found if we were politically committed.

As a direct result of the BCDDP, the American Cancer Society in 1988 joined with 12 national organizations, including the predominantly black National Medical Association, to issue specific guidelines for detecting breast cancer in asymptomatic women.

In certain cases of a strong family history of breast cancer, that is, cancer occurring before age 40, the first degree relatives (mother, daughters and sisters) have a 50% increased risk of early onset of breast cancer. For these women it is suggested that BSE begin at age fifteen and biennial mammography begin at age twenty, and then yearly at age thirty-five.**12**

By the same token young black women have proven to be at special risk.**13** For all black women, I suggest, in addition to early BSE, that mammography start at age 30 if there is any hint of nodules or lumpiness and continue on a yearly basis thereafter. Because of the density of the breast in these young women, mammography is 15 percent less effective. Though there is no doubt that cancers will be found, there will not be nearly as many cases as in older age groups. So the cost of each cancer found will be high. But think of the total number of productive years that can be added to the lives of those young women. It has been shown that discovering breast cancer early on is cost effective over the long run. See *Starting Mammography at 30 Something* later in this chapter.

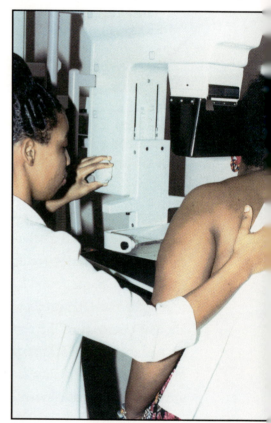

Fig. 6-3. Screening Mammography should be done at a facility certified by the American College of Radiology.

If every woman would take it upon herself to follow these guide-

A Needle in the Haystack

lines and urge friends and loved ones to also seek out screening programs, breast cancer would be discovered at a stage when the chance of cure is very likely.

Many clinics today, following the Guttman Institute lead, have opened their doors to earnestly seek out early breast cancer—at a reduced cost. But they are only seeing the tip of the iceberg, and many do not serve the needs of black and poor women because of their location, budgetary guidelines, etc. Another important factor to remember is that many black women don't even know these clinics exist.

Consequently, we must aggressively direct a keen dedicated offensive towards that population that appears to encompass the majority of women who succumb to breast cancer——the least informed. This would mean a special effort in the black community where "no information" and "mis-information" reign supreme.

Figures released by the National Cancer Institute indicate that during the five year period 1973 through 1977, the incidence of breast cancer increased 28 percent among black women compared to 18 percent among whites.[7]

There is a growing disparity in survival. Surveys conducted by the American Cancer Society in 1980 indicated that American black women are less exposed to cancer information than white women.[8] Lower income black women are less likely to perform breast self-examination. Blacks underestimate the prevalence of cancer and are less aware of cancer's warning signs. Although black and white women think of breast cancer when speaking generally of cancer only 30 percent of blacks had heard of a mammogram (x-ray) examination of the breast, compared to 53 percent of white women. Fifty-one percent of black women in the 1980 survey believed that exposing the cancer to air during surgery would cause spread of the malignancy. None of the white women questioned believed this myth.

The survey also showed that twice as many black women as white women voiced their desire not to be told they had cancer if it were true; and 59 percent of blacks believed that getting cancer is an automatic death sentence compared to only 36 percent of whites. Hopefully these misconceptions have been put to rest.

In 1988 health care screening specialists came together to discuss ways and means of getting more women screened for breast cancer. Like most of these "study groups" there was no real action because there was no real commitment for funding.9 Here we have one of the most readily diagnosed and treatable cancers in the spectrum being studied ad infinitum. The issue that can make a difference—funding for screening—is given lip service, talked to death and then put on the shelf until the next Talk-a-Thon. The last Talk-a-Thon, to my knowledge, was conducted by the Health Care Financing Administration in August, 1997. If history is any predictor, this latest talkfest will join the many previous pontifications on the dust heap of in-action. Another demonstration of paralysis of analysis.

Breast cancer screening should be an integral part of every health department in every community. If they can provide free immunizations for measles and mumps, they can provide mammography free of charge. If they can provide free Pap smears to detect early cervical cancer, then why not be as diligent in uncovering early breast cancer that kills three times as many black women before the age of thirty as cervical cancer.16 We need free mammograms on a grand scale. It is simply a matter of demand and creating the will without all the re-digestion of what we already know. The reason we don't have those screening facilities along with an overall adequate preventive health care system is because the politician is not responsive. Any time you reduce a health care system to a

---

GUIDELINES FOR BREAST CANCER DETECTION
(American Cancer Society)

1. Women 20 years of age and older should perform breast self-examination every month.

2. Women 20 to 40 years of age should have physical examination of the breast every three years, and women over 40 should have a physical examination of the breast every year. This should be done by a trained health provider.

3. Women at age 40 should have a baseline mammogram.*

4. Women between the ages of 40 and 50 should have a mammogram every two years.**

5. Women over age 50 should have a mammogram every year when feasible.

6. Women must consult their personal physician or clinic regarding the frequency of mammography in cases where there is a strong family history or other consideration.

*The original baseline recommended in 1977 was 35 years of age.

**In 1997 this recommendation was changed to every year.

A Needle in the Haystack

"for profit" managed care business, the needs of the patient and the compassion that instilled trust and respect in the health provider go out the window.

Politics is the ability to shape public policy and consensus through the legislative process. It's about wielding power and using compromise to get things done. It's an art form—a craft, a special talent. I don't have that talent; but I wouldn't be surprised if there is someone reading this chapter right now who does have that kind of organizational skill to pull it off. I'm sure, some of you readers know how to get things done. Politics means squeaking the wheel to get the oil. Some of you, I suspect, even have access to the ear of friends in high places.

If an articulate (or not so articulate) group of black women showed up at the local health department fired up and committed, on a regular basis there would be some action. In fact I bet if only a few choice sisters marched there would be a positive response.

But don't just start at the local health department. Go where the money is in the black community. Black entertainers, sports figures and talk show hosts would be eager to participate in funding screening programs, if only given the opportunity. Too many women are dying of breast cancer, unable to afford a screening mammogram. Let us not forget "...for whomsoever much is given of him shall much be required..." (Luke 12:48)

The answer is pure and simple. If you, the reader, want to find the needle in the haystack, then it's up to you to start digging. Knock on doors and get on the telephone. You know who to call.

Gear up for a massive ongoing effort of education and awareness in your community in order to somehow come to grips with this epidemic. Screening and education, and working in harmony, form a winning combination for maximum results. Do not get bound down in yet another *study of the problem*. Don't get trapped in yet another re-examination of what is already known.

There have been local efforts on the state level such as that in Wisconsin which showed that detection of breast cancer increased simply by instigating a breast cancer awareness program.**10** Similar programs in other parts of the country have also had some success.**11**

Until The Public Health Department catches up, private screening clinics must open their doors to the uninsured and the have-nots. In Montgomery, Alabama, some hospitals and private breast screening clinics open their doors to the uninsured once a year for little or no cost to the patient. Black women breast cancer survivors (Sistas CanSurvive Coalition) have organized and raised funds to provide mammography during October, targeted primarily to black indigent women. Encouraging women to get a mammogram is meaningless unless it is affordable and follow-up services are available. Black physicians have spear-headed the drive for funding. In Montgomery, Alabama and in many places people of goodwill are coming together in a redemptive spirit to uncover early, unsuspected breast cancer for eradication.

STARTING MAMMOGRAPHY AT 30 SOMETHING

Clinicians looking at the same information may disagree and indeed do disagree on how to interpret and apply that self-same information. For example the controversy regarding the age to start mammography is not settled. It is almost universally held that mammography screening in the 30-40 age bracket is not necessary, citing the rarity of breast cancer, the intolerable cost/effect ratio, the breast density of young women leading to unnecessary biopsies, the anxiety of mammography, and the concern that the x-ray may itself lead to breast cancer. Opponents to early mammography also rightly state that there is no uncontrovertible proof that early screening decreases mortality.

Let's examine each argument that favors mammography at a later age and omitting it at an earlier age, and then allow me to state my point of view or disagreement:

1. Spokespersons for the National Cancer Institute (NCI) continue to believe that there are no prospective randomized studies that indicate that mammography before age 50 impacts on breast cancer mortality. They only concede that lowering the age to 40 was a "political" decision (personal conversations), based more on emotion than science. Screening before age 50 *may* lower breast cancer mortality, but screening recommendations should be based on what is proven, they say.

The NCI opinion was based on a Canadian study that proved there was a statistical advantage to mammograms after age 50, but not before age 50.**17** However, the study has been highly criticized and found unreliable by authorities from several quarters.

Since that time, although no one study is large enough to provide the proof, combining the results of seven smaller studies revealed that there was an 18% lower mortality rate by virtue of screening women in the 40 to 49 year old age group. This 18% figure was based on screening every two to three years with only one view per breast. The reduced mortality would have been more impressive if the screening had been done on a yearly basis with two views per breast which is the standard today.**18-20**

Population based reports from the HIP Study and the BCDDP in which early breast cancer patients showed increased survival when diagnosed with mammography before age 50, has convinced the American Cancer Society and other medical groups that starting breast cancer screening at age 40 is reasonable.

To date there are no randomized clinical trials or population based studies regarding the value of mammography in mortality reduction for women specifically under age 40. Because the number of cases are too few to provide statistical analysis, it is not likely that a single trial study will ever be designed to answer that question for all to agree.

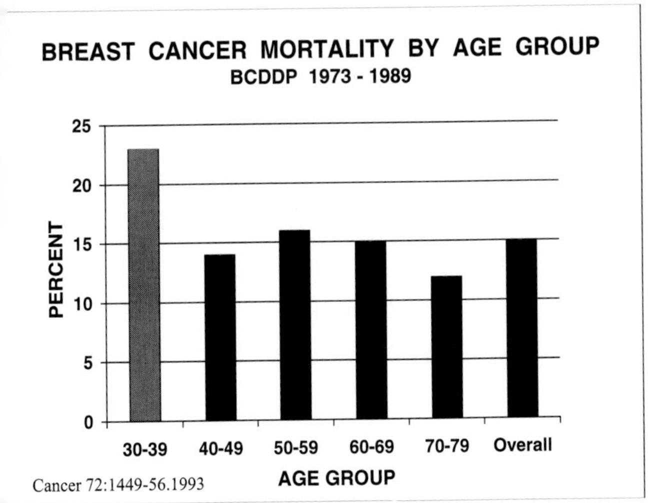

But we do agree that women younger than 35 have generally more aggressive cancers, are discovered when their cancer is large, and often extended beyond the breast. We do agree that after surgical treatment there is a higher recurrence rate in young women, and the mortality is higher than any other age group.**26,27**

It's not always necessary to wait for fool-proof studies to begin preventive measures. After

BREAST CANCER MORTALITY BY AGE GROUP
BCDDP 1973 - 1989

Cancer 72:1449-56.1993

Fig. 6-4. In the Breast Cancer Detection Demonstration Project, the highest mortality was in Women younger than 40.

all no one complains about Pap smear screening, colon cancer screening, prostate screening or even the breast self examination—none of which are based on randomized clinical trials. Yet most of us agree that it is reasonable to carry out those screenings.

Beginning mammography for many black women at age 40 may be too late. We see enough breast cancer in black women before age 40, often at Stage II and Stage III to wonder if a mammogram may have made a difference. In a study from Memorial Sloan Kettering Cancer Center it was found that screening women age 35 to 39 discovered 1.6 cancers per 1000 screened. Women in the 40-49 age group had 1.4 breast cancers discovered per 1000 screenees. The study concluded that probably just as much breast cancer will be found by screening women age 35-39 as women in the 40-49 age group and the cost is comparable. The investigators were careful to point out that a much larger number of women would be needed to verify this impression.[24]

According to the SEER Statistical Review **the age 40 is a time of sharp increase of breast cancer mortality in white women**. I suspect that is why the age 40 was chosen to begin mammography. The same SEER Review also reveals a different number for African-American women. **For black women the age of 35 is the point of comparable increase in mortality.**[22] This means, if we employ the same reasoning that we use for the general population, black women should at least be screened at age 35.

The truth of the matter is that even if a black woman dutifully follows screening guidelines designed for her white

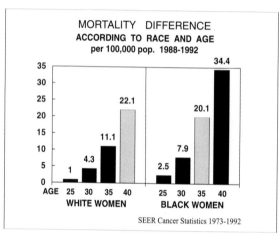

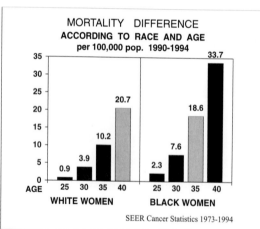

Fig. 6-5A, 5B. SEER Reports of 1992 and 1994 clearly show mortality for black women at 35 is comparable to white mortality at age 40.

A Needle in the Haystack

counterpart, her chance of survival will continue to be significantly less. **Guidelines written with white women in mind are simply not working for many black women.**

If all agree that mammography can detect breast cancer years before it can be felt, and that early detection directly affects the chance of survival, then for black women it may be time to re-think the issues according to statistics that affect black women rather than the general population i.e. white women.

2. Breast Self Examination should be the mainstay of detecting early breast cancer before the age of 40 because the breasts are dense, and breast cancer will not be detected in 10-15% of dense breasts.

The sensitivity of mammography in detecting early breast cancer in young women is not related to the density of the breast when using modern-day mammography x-ray machines. Decreased sensitivity is related to family history of breast cancer and size of tumor. On the other hand, women, older than 50, regardless of their menopausal status ,breast density if present, does indeed decrease sensitivity of the mammogram.**30**

Nevertheless, detection machines are getting better all the time. We now have high definition gray scale digitally enhanced computerized mammography. We now know that double reading can increase accuracy up to 15%. We shall soon have the RODEO and SPECT imaging techniques. See Chapter 3.

A woman with dense breasts needs to be doubly vigilant with increased mammography studies, not less. It has been shown in the BCDDP studies that breast density over 50% increases the chance of breast cancer, and a 75% increased density leads to a five-fold increase in breast cancer whether the woman is premenopausal or post menopausal.**25**

If you are concerned that mammography will miss a cancer, you must also realize that breast self-examination (BSE) will miss at least 50% of tumors even by the hands of trained clinicians. And, if indeed found by palpation, the cancer may have been present for several years. I believe that a major reason why black women are diagnosed with advanced disease so much is that mammography is not started at an early age.

3. It is not cost effective to provide mammograms before age 40.

The incidence of breast cancer under age 40 is 94.5/100,000 population for white women and 109.3 for black women. When you compare the incidence of women ages 40-49 (443.3 white women and 398.5 black women)**22**, one might believe that since there are fewer cases in the younger age, the cost of screening would not justify the number of cancers found. However, there is a humane side to the equation that defines preventive medical care that must not be forgotten.

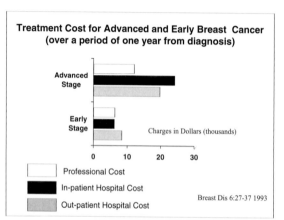

Even if we put aside the humane question, it was reported in 1993 that finding breast cancer early on saved dollars in the long run.**23** The authors assumed that 25% of women age 25-75 had mammograms. Of the breast cancers discovered, one year of treatment for an advanced breast cancer patient would be 2.5 times as costly as the treatment for early stage cancer. These figures do not include medication costs, extra medical office visits, fees for additional specialists and ancillary care, employment disability costs, cost for palliative treatment, and lost wages.

Fig. 7. Cost effectiveness is best when Breast Cancer is found is found at an early Stage.

4. Screening mammograms before age 40 causes anxiety and false positive studies leading to needless biopsies.

No one can disagree that obtaining a mammogram can be a moment of high anxiety, and that finding a suspicious shadow can unleash the dogs of fear and despair. At the same time to ignore the enemy is not the answer. See Chapter 8. The majority of biopsies are negative for cancer. But negative does not mean the biopsy was needless. A biopsy cannot be deemed needless if there is any legitimate suspicion. A pre-cancerous lesion may be found, and such findings mean added risk requiring heightened vigilance. With fewer open biopsies and more needle biopsies being done, I suspect the fear of breast scarring and prolonged disability following the biopsy will be less problematic.

A Needle in the Haystack

5. The mammogram may pose a danger of radiation exposure which may cause cancer.

The effects of radiation exposure are cumulative and the effects may not be manifest for ten to twenty years. Thirty-five years ago when x-rays machines were less sophisticated and xeroradiography was also being done with significant radiation exposure, there was legitimate concern and a rationale to limit mammography. Since 1994 the American College of radiology has made strides in setting standards regarding the quality of mammogram centers and the dose of radiation that would be acceptable. Studies have shown that the average radiation dose at certified mammogram facilities for two views of each breast would total 0.4 rad (2.0 mGy).**29**

If screening began at age 40 and continued on an annual basis until age 75, radiation induced breast cancer would be virtually zero. If mammography began at age 35 and continued annually until age 75, the benefit/risk ratio would be extremely favorable. If a million women are screened 800 to 4,000 cancers will be found with the potential of inducing only 3 cancers.**28**

These figures are based on incidence in the general population. Since it is known that for black women there is relatively more breast cancer in younger women and the life expectancy is less than 75 years, the benefit to risk ratio for black women should be higher when starting mammography at 35. In any case, with these low exposures, the remote chance of radiation induced breast cancer should not dissuade women from early mammography.

In these times of impersonalized health care being foisted upon us, I find October, breast cancer awareness month, a time to rally the community to finding the needle in the haystack.

If an early cancer is found, then the practice and art of medicine is somehow justified—again it becomes a noble pursuit. Being a physician or health care provider must be more than just making a good living. Like Arthur Ashe said: "Getting makes a living, …giving makes a life". Black leaders in the medical profession must join others in getting across a message that is crystal clear. The public and the politicians must understand:

Breast cancer can be detected early. Discovery can be both practical and cost efficient. Through monthly breast self-examination, periodic medical examination, and mammography screening—incredulous though it may seem, the needle in the haystack can be found!

———————

As black women take on more of the responsibility of their personal health, the question of participating in clinical trials must be addressed. In the next chapter I shall discuss clinical trials and their importance in discovering new methods to combat and control breast cancer.

CHAPTER SEVEN

N THE SHADOW OF TUSKEGEE
Clinical Trials and Black Women

*p*lainly stated, a "clinical trial" is an experiment using human beings to find the best treatment for a particular disease, or improve on the accepted standard of care. The trial is conducted by comparing two groups of patients. One group is given a standard accepted treatment and the second group is given some new drug or treatment method. After a period of time the groups are compared. The group that shows the best response is assumed to have received the superior treatment and that treatment is then accepted as the standard of care.

Since complications and side effects of a new drug may be unpredictable, every patient that participates in a clinical trial demonstrates a courage that we must respect. Nonetheless, if monitored appropriately with safeguards in place, clinical trial participation is generally safe and poses an intriguing option for many patients.

Black women are well represented in treatment trials, but the numbers are lacking in the prevention and screening trials.

It may be that black women are not being actively recruited by clinical investigators for clinical trials. Or it may be that black women are hesitant because in times past, the necessary safeguards for black participants were not always in place. Between the years 1932 and 1972 the United States Public Health Service conducted so-called clinical studies in Tuskegee, Alabama. Hundreds of black men with syphilis were recruited ostensibly to receive treatment for their disease. The truth of the matter is that those men got no treatment even after Penicillin was known to be curative. The hidden agenda was simply to observe all the stages of syphilis until death. The Tuskegee Study was not an ethical study. In fact, it was the longest nontherapeutic experiment on human beings in medical history.

What happened in Tuskegee is even more dastardly when one considers the Nurenberg Code of the 1940's that grew out of the Nurenberg trials of Nazi war criminals. The Code that was drafted affirmed the dignity of the human being involved as a research subject. It stated that all humans should be assured that they would not be exploited and that strict ethical standards would be observed.

Nevertheless in the Tuskegee experiment, begun in 1932, the lofty ideals of the Nurenberg Code were ignored. Black men were reduced to the status of guinea pigs until 1972, courtesy of the United States Public Health Service.

Some sixty years later, a few elderly men who were participants, and scores of relatives of the deceased victims, received an apology from President Clinton, speaking on behalf of the nation. The meager class action suit won earlier by the NAACP would be small consolation for this act of barbarism.

That bit of history makes it difficult to recruit black women to breast cancer clinical trials. As a result of the Tuskegee debacle, I suspect, clinical trials in the black community will be uniformly shunned by many for the foreseeable future. Black folks, with good reason, are suspicious of their government and the medical profession when it comes to clinical testing.

At the same time it is patently clear that African-Americans should participate in modern clinical trials to advance the body of knowledge of proper health care. Only through this method has it been shown that prostate cancer, prominent in black males, can be treated by other means rather than castration. Only through this method has it been shown that conservative surgery as opposed to mastectomy can be equally effective in breast cancer cure.

Clinical trials of today are carefully monitored. If a treatment appears to be unrewarding or harmful it is halted.

Ultimately, improved health care comes from pulling down barriers to access, bolstering preventive measures, and treating the patient with compassion and respect. But expanding our knowledge base is equally as important. And one way of increasing our knowledge is through clinical trials.

To that end the National Cancer Institute has sponsored the Minority-Based Community Clinical Oncology Program [MBCCOP] to foster black participation in institutions which serve a large minority population. Through clinical trials we can test the merits of mammography as opposed to newer imaging techniques in detecting cancers in young women. In this way clinical preventive trials may very well be an important factor in affecting the appalling breast cancer mortality statistics among young black women. As mentioned elsewhere in this book, present day screening guidelines are not working for black women. Statistics point to the fact that black women tend to contract breast cancer at an earlier age. Hence a preventive screening clinical trial that answers the question about early mammograms vis-a-vis other screening techniques for black women should be based on the black breast cancer experience, not on the experience of the general population. Black women must not be allowed to continue teetering on the fringes of the health care delivery system—playing the role of catch-as-catch-can.

Less than 0.5% of current researchers engaged in clinical trials are African-American. Many in that select group have come together to champion the cause of clinical trials in the black community. They have formed an organization called the Society of Cancer Researchers Advocating Therapeutic Excellence for Special Populations [SOCRATES] that serves as an overseer of clinical trials. Their purpose is to assure participating African-Americans that a particular study is not only relevant, but that it is also carefully monitored and due precautions are observed.[4] This overseer role should be spearheaded at the local level by community leaders. Every clinical trial based at any medical center in this country must have built-in oversight conducted by a board made up partially of local people from the population being studied. It is called the Institutional Review Board. We must not depend on the loose structure of SOCRATES to shoulder the responsibility of oversight. The focus should be on local people keeping watch over their own.

In view of the Tuskegee Syphilis Study, it will take the combined effort of SOCRATES and primary black health providers along with community leaders on the Institutional Review Board to educate the black populace on the benefits of clinical trials, and to assure them that oversight is mandatory by law. The black media, the black church and black civic groups must join together in an effort to recruit black women to breast cancer clinical trials.

Since women must be referred by their doctor to a clinical trial, the black doctor, in many instances, stands as the gatekeeper with the responsibility of directing patients to ongoing clinical trials.[1]

Before a drug or new treatment method can be considered for approval by the Food and Drug Administration (FDA) it must undergo three phases of scrutiny:

Phase I Trial

Only after extensive studies in the laboratory and using animal experimentation, Phase I clinical trials using healthy human volunteers may be started. Phase I investigations in humans are concerned with assessing a drug's safety at various dosage levels. Toxicity and side effects are recorded. Because of some inherent dangers, a relatively small number of participants are used, usually 20 to 50—certainly not more than 100. The study determines how the drug is absorbed, metabolized and excreted. This initial Phase is conducted over several months. About 70 percent of drugs tested in this Phase go on to the next step.

In a different context, a desperately ill patient considered terminal

---

QUESTIONS TO ASK BEFORE PARTICIPATING IN A CLINICAL TRIAL

1. What is the purpose of the trial? Exactly what question(s) will the trial answer?

2. What are the risks involved?

3. How will the patient's safety be monitored?

4. What happens if the patient is somehow harmed by the trial?

5. Can the patient withdraw from the trial at any time for any reason or no reason without penalty.

6. Is there a payment to the patient in exchange for participation? (In Phase I trials remuneration is common.)

7. Is there any charge for medical care and medication?

8. What are the possible benefits to the participant?

9. How long will the trial last?

In the Shadow of Tuskegee

may be offered an untried treatment to determine safe dosage levels and other characteristics of the drug. A patient must understand that enrolling in a Phase I trial is designed primarily to learn more about the characteristics of the new drug, not necessarily to provide medical treatment.

Phase II Trial

If a drug was found to be safe in Phase I trials, it must next be tested for efficacy. In other words, does the new drug work, and is it a better alternative than the standard treatment?

In the Phase II studies several hundred patients must be enrolled in order to support statistical analyses.

Usually neither the patient nor the researcher knows which patient received the new drug. In this way bias is curtailed and the FDA can better assess the merits of the new treatment. Only 30 percent of new drugs pass Phase I and Phase II trials.

Phase III Trial

This Phase requires several thousand participants, divided into groups to compare the new treatment(s) against the standard care. Data is collected and participants are observed over several years. During this period a greater understanding of the efficacy, side effects and cost benefit ratio can be achieved. Phase III is the final step in determining whether a new drug should be included in future treatment protocols. It is now ready to be submitted to the FDA for approval.

Phase IV Trial

In this late post-acceptance phase, a drug's long term effects are studied. Often the new drug is compared with other standard treatments and combined with other standard treatments in search of enhanced benefit. The effect on quality of life and cost benefit is delineated.

———

Studies have shown that the general care is superior to medical care outside the clinical trial setting. Patients gain access to new treatments before the general population often to their benefit. There seems to be little question that longevity is enhanced by Phases II/III clinical trial participation.**2**

The Sickle-cell Trial is a case in point. Researchers, attempting to find a better method of controlling the effects of sickle-cell anemia, discovered that an experimental method being tested worked so well that the clinical trial was halted, and all patients received the new treatment. This trial has proven to be a breakthrough in the treatment of sickle-cell disease.

Before any study gets underway we must enlist the support of primary health providers, doctors and clinics in the black community.**3** Through primary health resources we can recruit a critical mass of black women for clinical trials.

It would seem extremely unlikely that a Tuskegee fiasco will ever be repeated now that all clinical trials are subjected to the scrutiny of an Institutional Review Board. The Board is composed of health professionals of the sponsoring institution along with community lay persons. Black organizations must demand a place on these local Boards and be directly involved in the overseeing of the clinical trials. The Tuskegee escapade could not have happened if such a Board had been in place.

In Appendix D there is a listing of some of the Clinical Trials going on in 1997-98 regarding Breast Cancer. This is just the tip of the iceberg. The National Cancer Institute's PDQ database is the most comprehensive database on clinical trials with over 150 clinical trials listed pertaining to breast cancer. Call the hotline at the National Cancer Institute (1-800-4-CANCER) to learn more about clinical trials in your area; or you can dial Cancer Fax at 301 402 587.

———

Once breast cancer cancer is uncovered, women must have some information regarding Classification and Staging. Treatment decisions are based on such knowledge. If the patient is expected to participate in her care she must have a body of information for consideration and perusal. In the next chapter information is provided that can afford a point of reference to initiate discussion and questions with your health provider.

In the Shadow of Tuskegee

CHAPTER EIGHT

O NEWS IS GOOD NEWS, RIGHT? WRONG! Know the Enemy to Survive

*Y*ou and I fear cancer because it may bring suffering and death. In fact we tend to deny any sickness as long as possible. We run from the notion of illness like the Boston marathon. It's just human nature to avoid realities that may be unpleasant. As for a check-up. Forget it. We don't want any blood tests or even a chest x-ray. Who wants bad news? No news is good news. Right? And so we wait for pain or some disability to goad us to the doctor; and then we hope for some miracle or a good report to speed us on our way, to await the next signal of pain.

Most physicians, like me, are just like you. We're all in the same bag. Some doctors drink too much, eat too much, and some of us are still smoking. We doctors fail to get check ups, too—including me.

But just for a moment let me tell you what I think is right, not what I necessarily do. If you're walking around knowing you have a lump in your breast, you should seek medical help. However, if you're putting it off, because of fear, you're not the only one. You've got lots of company. Seventy-five percent of American women rank breast cancer as their number one health fear as noted by The Opinion Research Corporation of Princeton, New Jersey. Fear is a natural reaction to breast cancer or any lump in the breast. And it's hard to go in for a mammogram. It's easier to put it off. How many black men over 40 actually get a rectal exam and a blood study to check for prostate trouble periodically as recommended? The average man, I suspect, waits until he can not urinate before he gets a prostate checkup.

Anyway, who wants bad news? No news is good news. Right? Perhaps not. Ignorance may be bliss, but when it comes to breast cancer, or prostate cancer for that matter, we may miss an opportunity for cure, simply by not acting responsibly. Sometimes bad news can turn out okay if it is dealt with in a timely manner. So do your best to take control and direct old man fear to trigger you towards some positive action.

A positive response would be to learn as much as you can about breast cancer now. Know your enemy! Learn how breast cancer can be controlled, and even cured in its early stages. Check with the Public Health Department in your community. Call your doctor or clinic and inquire about available information. A number of pamphlets can be obtained through the Department of Health and Human Services; and the American Medical Association will provide cancer information at a nominal cost. No news is not good news. It's ignorance.

Another good source of information, mostly free for the asking, is provided through the local chapter of the American Cancer Society.
Films and speakers are available for groups to stimulate discussion and answer questions. There is too much misinformation circulating in our community. These agencies will welcome your questions and input in designing a presentation for your church group or club.

Black women breast cancer survivors groups may be available in your community. They represent an excellent source of information. If you are interested in forming a local group to gain information and/or spread the message, call one of the groups in Chapter 10 or Appendix B for direction.

For diagnosis and treatment it may be advisable to seek out a comprehensive cancer clinic if you live in a metropolitan area. These clinics are part of every university medical center, and free-standing breast centers are springing up in cities and towns across the nation. Be sure the facility has state of the art equipment and a certified radiologist to interpret the x-rays.

The Office of Cancer Communications, National Cancer Institute, Bethesda, MA, would be able to direct you to a center near your home. Other sources to explore include The Susan G Komen Breast Cancer Foundation, or The National Women's Health Network in Washington, DC. See Appendix A for an up-to-date listing of resources.

Every woman should develop the capacity to suspect the breast cancer intruder in the very early months before distant spread. With some familiarity with the different stages of breast cancer and even the micro-scopic patterns as they pertain to prognosis, a patient can help herself towards wellness by appreciating the facts of her case; and thus be more inclined to cooperate with the treatment program outlined by her doctor. Most physicians agree that breast cancer is a disease in which the patient is expected to participate in learning about the types of breast cancer and the implications for care.

The following discussion is included to help answer some ques-tions for readers who wish a more in-depth discussion. You may find it too detailed and you may wish to skip over it and go on to Chapter 9—The Battle Plan.

HISTOLOGY (CELLULAR PATTERN)

Every type of breast cancer can be classified by its unique pattern of malignant cells as viewed through the microscope. Each type of cancer has its own distinctive growth idiosyncrasy that bears on treatment options and ultimate survival. Two breast cancers of the same size may have entirely different poten-tials for local extension and dissemination. In one case the breast cancer may be aggressive and spreads early while in another case the cancer may tend to develop slowly and have less propensity to metasta-size even when the pri-mary tumor is fairly bulky.1

Dr Edwin Fisher of the University of Pittsburgh Medical

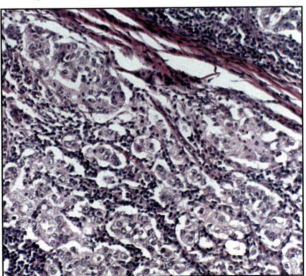

Fig. 8-1. Infiltrating Ductal Carcinoma. The light gray-blue cells are cancer. This 48 year-old black woman had never had a screening mammogram. There was one positive node in the axilla. She received a modified radical mastectom-followed by radiation and chemotherapy.

School showed that the ultimate prognosis depends, not only on the extent of spread of the cancer when first detected, but also on the cellular type involved. He named six major cellular types that have differing survival implications.

Infiltrating Ductal

Fifty percent of all breast cancers can be recognized as Infiltrating Ductal. In some series as many as 75 percent are classified as Infiltrating Ductal. If we disregard the extent of spread and look at all cases with this cellular pattern, we find that 60 percent will not be cured.

Lobular Invasive

The Lobular Invasive type on the other hand, accounts for only 6 percent of the cancer cell types and the prognosis is better. 30 percent will be treatment failures.

Lobular Carcinoma in Situ

Lobular Carcinoma in Situ cancer (LCIS) has only been known for the past fifty years. As mentioned in Chapter 4 this lesion is not a cancer, but a clear marker that cancer will occur in 20-30 percent of cases. There is no clear marker on the mammogram and it cannot be felt on physical examination. Generally it is found by accident when suspicious calcifications are biopsied. LCIS may then be viewed by the microscope, although it is not actually associated with the calcification. It almost always occurs in premenopausal women and can be treated by simple observation with yearly mammograms if there are no other risk factors. Cancer may develop in either breast. The opposite breast (contralateral) may also be involved.

Some surgeons believe that simple mastectomy of the involved breast and close observation of the contralateral breast is preferable treatment, while others advised bilateral mastectomy.2 Recently, this approach has been questioned, since the chance of breast cancer increases only 1percent per year for the first ten years after discovery. I advise close observation.

Ductal Carcinoma in Situ (DCI).

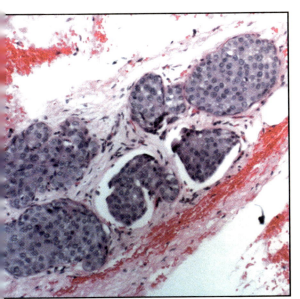

ig. 8-2. Ductal Carcinoma in Situ. The urple cells are cancer confined at this oint, but will eventually invade.

Although this classification was not part of Dr Fisher's original paper, it is important to mention at this time since it may be confused with Lobular Carcinoma in Situ. DCI is a true cancer that has not invaded the surrounding tissue although there may be hidden invasion in 20 percent of cases. They present as nipple discharge or large palpable lesions. About 20 percent of breast cancers are DCI and are detected often by discovering calcifications on mammography. The chance of invasion is 60 percent; hence most surgeons would suggest mastectomy for large cancers, or lumpectomy with adequate margins for smaller lesions, followed by radiation. Axillary dissection is usually not done for DCI.**10**

It has been found that DCI as well as LCIS are more common in African American women. This has implications for heightened vigilance particularly in the younger women.**11**

Medullary, Mucinous, or Tubular

Approximately 5 percent of all cases of breast cancer will be either the Medullary, Mucinous or Tubular type with a moderate prognosis. The failure rate is 27 percent, discounting the stage. In early cases the prognosis is excellent with less than a 7 percent treatment failure. It should be noted that medullary carcinoma is more common in black women.**8**

Combination Group

A final histologic cancer type cited by Dr Fisher is the Combination group. In this situation more than one histologic pattern is found in the same cancer. These are mostly Infiltrating Ductal and Tubular, or Infiltrating Ductal and Lobular (invasive) combinations. Occasionally,

Mucinous and other rare types are associated with Infiltrating Ductal. The treatment failure rate in the Combination group is 25 percent.

Paget's Disease and Inflammatory Breast Cancer

Two unusual breast cancers, classified under Infiltrating Ductal, should be emphasized since they can be readily detected. They are Paget's Disease, and Inflammatory Cancer.

Paget's Disease is first detected as a rash over the nipple that slowly creeps out over the areola. It looks like an ordinary irritation. After a week or so of home remedies, a patient may visit the family doctor or a dermatologist who may prescribe a cream for the rash that, of course, doesn't work. In disgust the woman may disregard her return appointment to the dermatologist and seek out another physician after several weeks. That doctor may prescribe an antibiotic ointment, wasting precious time. The wiser patient would have either returned to the dermatologist or informed the second physician that creams and ointments had not helped after a few weeks of trial. Undoubtedly, with this history either physician would have suggested a biopsy under local anesthesia. A tiny fragment of skin the size of a pin-head would tell the story. Paget's Disease represents only 2.5 percent of all breast cancers. The typical rash is usually found before a tumor is palpable under the nipple. If treated early about 70 percent will be cured.

Inflammatory breast cancer which is uniformly fatal is extremely rare. It begins as a dusky redness in the dependent part of the breast and simulates mastitis or the inflamed breast of the nursing mother. Although the cancer is incurable life can be extended with early therapy.

Comedo Cancer

Another term you may hear that describes a breast cancer is comedo carcinoma, usually associated with the infiltrating ductal type. Comedo means there is an accumulation of cancer cells in the ducts with severe local infiltration of the neighboring tissue that indicates a worse prognosis.

———

Not only cellular type but the capacity to infiltrate into surrounding tissue affects prognoses. If veins and lymph channels near the primary cancer are clogged with cancer cells, the recurrent rate is high. Also the size of the lesion is significant. Dr Fisher found that cancers 5 centimeters or larger have metastasized when first discovered, even if the lymph nodes seem to be uninvolved.

Location of the tumor in the breast has implications for the direction of spread. Most cancers occur in the upper outer quadrant with spread into the lymph nodes of the axilla. Tumors that arise in the medial half of the breast also tend to metastasize to the axilla. However, a significant percent will spread medially and infiltrate the internal mammary nodes along the breast bone.

STAGING BREAST CANCER

The most often used method of classifying breast cancer is according to the size of the tumor and the extent of spread to regional lymph nodes and beyond these confines.[4] Also, to be considered is whether the lesion involves the skin or has penetrated to be fixed to the underlying muscle. With this information one is able to stage the cancer according to the TNM System (Tumor size, Nodes, Metastasis). This TNM System was devised in 1973 by the American Joint Committee for Cancer Staging and End Results (AJCCSER). There are four Stages in the TNM System and the prognosis worsens with an increase in the Stage number.

In recent years the TNM System has been criticized for its short-

---

THE TNM STAGING SYSTEM according to the AJCCSER

STAGE I T=Breast tumor of any size up to 5 centimeters, minimal skin involvement, no muscle or chest wall attachment. N=No axillary nodes palpable. M=No distant metastasis.

STAGE II T=Same as Stage I. N=One or more nodes palpable in the axilla. M=No distant metastasis.

STAGE III T=Breast tumor over 5 centimeters. N=Same as Stage II plus one or more of the following: Skin ulceration, skin edema, pectoral muscle attachment, nodes fixed in the axilla

STAGE IV Spread of cancer beyond the axilla (distant metastasis to bone, lung, brain, liver, etc).

TNM STAGING CLASSIFICATION
according to the IUAC

STAGE 0 T=Lobular Carcinoma in Situ or Intraductal Carcinoma in Situ

STAGE I T=Breast tumor of any size up to 2 centimeters, minimal skin involvement, no muscle or chest wall attachment. N=No axillary nodes palpable. M=No distant metastasis.

STAGE IA T=Breast tumor 5 millimeters or smaller.
STAGE IB T=Breast tumor over 5 millimeters to 2 centimeters.

STAGE IIA T=No evidence of tumor in breast. N=One or more nodes paplpable in the axilla. M=No distant metastasis.
STAGE IIB T=Breast tumor between 2 and 5 centimeters. N=One or more nodes palpable in the axilla. M=No distant metastasis.
STAGE IIB T=Breast tumor larger than 5 centimeters. N=No axillary nodes. M=No distant metastasis.

STAGE IIIA T=No evidence of tumor in breast. N=One or more nodes in the axilla fixed and not movable. M=No distant metastasis.
STAGE IIIA T=Breast tumor less than 2 centimeters. N= One or more nodes in the axilla fixed and not movable. M=No distant metastasis.
STAGE IIIA T=Breast tumor between 2 and 5 centimeters. N=One or more nodes in the axilla fixed and not movable. M=No distant metastasis.
STAGE IIIA T=Breast tumor greater than 5 centimeters. N=One or more nodes in axilla freely movable. Or one or more nodes fixed and not movable.
STAGE IIIB T=Tumor of any size with direct extension to the skin or chest wall N=Nodes present or not present in axilla. M=No distant metastasis.

STAGE IV Spread of cancer beyond the axilla (distant metastasis to bone, lung, brain, liver, etc).

No News is Good News, Right? Wrong!

comings and inaccuracies. The International Union Against Cancer (IUAC), a world body of oncologists, has refined the system and it is the current system that most clinicians employ when discussing the Stage of breast cancer.9 Although microscopic evaluation and estrogen receptor status and other more sophisticated tests are important prognostic indicators, TNM Staging is often used to help decide treatment options and to determine prognosis.

Regardless of admitted imperfection, Staging serves as a useful guide in designing treatment protocols and answering questions concerning prognosis. For example, a patient with Stage I with treatment has an 80 percent chance of surviving ten years or more. A woman in Stage II can expect a 60 percent survival rate at ten years, while a Stage III cancer patient would expect only a 30 percent chance of living free of disease for ten years. These figures can improve depending on the cellular type of cancer involved. Life can also be extended for months and years through various treatment modalities.

I can't expect you to remember all the cellular types of breast cancer. The pathologist (physician who looks at the tissue under the microscope) knows the cellular types and your surgeon also has some familiarity with the subject. Many surgeons insist on seeing the microscopic sections and having the pathologist point out the highlights of the cancer that bear on prognosis.

This information provided here will assist you to ask specific questions of your doctor. If a breast biopsy shows the cancer enemy lurking along a duct or infiltrating the normal tissue, inquire about the cell type that was found and what that means with regards to treatment and prognosis. What was the size of the tumor? Over 5 centimeters? Under 2 centimeters? What section of the breast was the cancer located and were any lymph nodes positive for cancer? And what does all this mean in terms of survival?

There is data suggesting that the location of the cancer in the breast, whether it be near the breast bone or the armpit, has little or no bearing on the prognosis or curability. Nevertheless, some investigators believe that cancers near the midline require radiation directed to that site. Ask your doctor his understanding of this controversy.

There is also the question of blood type and prognosis. British doctors reported in 1970 that women with breast cancer with a blood type of B or AB had a significantly higher incidence and recurrence rate than women with blood type A or O. More recently investigators have not found such a relationship.[5,6]

You may also wish to know if the cancer is estrogen-receptor positive and/or progesterone-receptor positive? These receptor tests on the cancerous tissue that is removed were discussed in Chapter 3. Also be sure a DNA Histogram is done on any biopsy tissue. You don't have to know the definition of aneuploidy or the meaning of oncogenes, but ask your doctor to help you know your prognosis—to give you some idea of the aggressiveness of the cancer.[7]

Even if you can't remember the details of the tests and tumor types, ask anyway. What kind of tumor do I have? What were the results of the DNA histogram and the ER and PR tests? How does this affect my prognosis and the treatment program? What are my options regarding chemotherapy? And what about Tamoxifen? Your surgeon will know you're concerned and will answer all questions in terms that you can understand. In fact he'll work a little harder on your behalf. You've got to know the cancer enemy to enhance your opportunity for survival; and you must have information to participate in decisions of treatment.

On the other hand many women have little desire to know the details of the disease or the outline of any proposed treatment regimen. Maybe the only news that interests you is simply some indication of your chances of cure. You may want to leave the details to your doctor and his discussions with your family. You may need time to sort things out, to regroup so to speak. Most women, in my experience, eventually come to terms with the disease; and, at some point, expect and appreciate an explanation of treatment alternatives based on the Stage of disease and the histologic type. But everyone at her own pace and her own needs.

———

Becoming familiar with the major aspects of the breast cancer will not only help you to understand the danger, but will stress the need for an early counterattack. In the next chapter I will turn to that counterattack.

CHAPTER NINE

THE BATTLE PLAN
What is the Best Treatment for Breast Cancer Today?

a carefully conceived plan of action is the key to success no matter what the occasion. Whether it's Thanksgiving turkey with all the trimmings or the wedding of the year with all the frills, any successful event requires forethought and planning.

Team sports are good examples where planning means winning. All teams study their opponents and map out a plan for winning. They call it the game plan. In football, with all the brute physical contact, I believe it is really a battle plan. It's flexible and the coach can change it on the spot to cope with changing circumstances of the game.

Obviously, the battle plan to control and eradicate disease also continues to change in light of new medical discoveries and innovative technology. Careful planning and attention to the game plan have led to marvelous victories in the medical field; and over the years many dread diseases in this country, such as small pox, measles, and polio, have been controlled or eliminated. Breakthroughs in treating certain cancers, such as childhood leukemia have also been achieved in our time.

In spite of these advances in medical sophistication, the battles to conquer major cancers, such as lung, colon, breast, pancreas, and prostate are often tedious with too few victories to record.

In this chapter let us examine how the battle against breast cancer is faring. Are there any victories we can point to? Are there any victories on the horizon? Let's review the different treatment strategies promulgated by today's experienced clinicians.

For a long time we attacked breast cancer like the early football players, sloshing through the mud with the snug helmet and baggy pants, with only a make-shift game plan. We were akin to the Roman legions with only spear and shield, waging war on breast cancer by radical, mutilating surgery.

Ah, but times have changed. Football has become a safer sport with advances in equipment and technique. The basic weapons of war and defense are no longer the Roman spear and shield; and the battle plan to control breast cancer has also changed and continues to evolve.

The strategy today in the struggle against breast cancer calls for painstaking development and testing of new anti-cancer weapons. Many years are spent testing and comparing treatment programs; and when there are variations of many therapies and several combinations of complicated treatment protocols, defining the best therapy is often imprecise.

Nevertheless, we have come some distance in recent decades in changing our general philosophy on how breast cancer should be attacked. It is now believed to be a systemic disease, almost from the very beginning, rather than localized. There has also been advances in our knowledge of how the body's natural defenses operate, and how those defense systems can be enhanced.

However, there remains a remnant of personal bias and passion for entrenched ideas that occasionally confuse the issue when defining the optimal treatment plan. Statistics have been used to reflect foregone conclusions. Doctors quoting the same statistics have drawn diametrically opposing conclusions. Disraeli, the nineteenth century English statesman, once said, "There are liars, damn liars, and statistics." Here's an example. A study at the Guy Hospital in London compared the radical mastectomy to local excision and radiation.[1] The five-year survival favored the radical mastectomy in Stage II cases and was widely quoted by proponents favoring radical surgery. The ten-year survival, however, showed no statistical difference and that figure, naturally was quoted by the radiation enthusiasts. Nevertheless, through research and carefully planned clinical trials, and with less emotion and bias, new insight in preferred attacks have been defined.

At the turn of the century the battle cry of most surgeons in America was, "Cut out as much as you can." Of course, there were dissenters. The French surgeon, Matas, in 1900, Dr. George Crile, Sr., in the 1920's, and Dr. Keynes of England, in the 1930's, were convinced that a lesser surgery was adequate; but their ideas fell on deaf ears.[2] The notion that radical surgery was the only way to control and cure breast cancer was firmly planted in the American surgical dogma; and the vast majority of surgeons followed this dictum in lock-step for the next 75 years.

Radiation to treat breast cancer came on the scene in the 1930's and 1940's. As you might imagine x-ray machines were little more than simple radiation emitters in the early days. The correct radiation dose was unknown and the results were unpredictable and often tragic.

About the same time it was observed that estrogens helped some post-menopausal women and castration prolonged life in a minority of younger women before the menopause. However, there was no way to predict who would be helped.

Next came Dr. Huggin's work in the 1950's, demonstrating the value of adrenalectomy and hypophysectomy (removal of the adrenal and pituitary glands).[3] This new battle plan, however, was compromised by significant morbidity and death.

Finally, chemotherapy was introduced in the 1960's with its own set of complications such as hair loss, severe nausea, bone marrow depression and even death. Subsequent combinations of these drugs have been used to advantage and some lengthening of life has been reported.

Various investigators pleaded for radiation early in the battle. Others decried radiation in favor of surgery only; and there were many protagonists advocating different forms of surgery and combinations of surgery and radiation. Finally, some proponents spoke of a melding of radiation, chemotherapy, hormones, and surgery. These debates often generated more heat than light.

Even today the battle plan is still being focused and redefined; and I suspect it will continue in a state of flux while various clinical trials come to fruition.

Presently, treatment decisions must be designed for the individual woman with the best information available. Treatment, as well as screening, for African American women must be based on information gleaned from studying the African American population.

In over half the breast cancer cases found in black women, cancer has already spread beyond the confines of the breast when the diagnosis is made.[4] It can be detected in the axilla, the lung, the bone, the brain, and the liver. Surgery and radiation can only hope to control the primary site and local lymph node spread. The body's inherent immune system usually deals effectively with microscopic dissemination. However, immunity can quickly be overwhelmed and the patient rendered unable to deal with a large host of tumor cells. At that point chemotherapy may be helpful but not curative. Chemotherapy should not be used too soon since investigators have shown that drugs used prematurely can impair the immune system to the patient's detriment.

For the reader who is not inclined to know the details in the development of various treatment methods, please turn to the segment, THE BATTLE PLAN TODAY, found towards the end of this chapter. However, for those wanting an overview of how we got to where we are today in treating breast cancer, the following paragraphs should be helpful.

THE HALSTEAD RADICAL MASTECTOMY

In 1894 William Halstead of the Johns Hopkins Medical Center in Baltimore, devised the radical mastectomy—the same operation thousands of surgeons world-wide have performed over the decades.[5] The nipple and a large segment of skin along with the entire breast and underlying muscle on the chest wall (pectoralis major and pectoralis minor), plus the fat containing lymph nodes of the axilla were excised en bloc, that is altogether, as a single specimen. See Chapter Two.

Emphasis was placed on the en bloc dissection because of the penetration and contiguous spread of these neglected cases that were presented to Dr Halstead in the early years of the 20th century. Halstead believed that cutting through the specimen would possibly spread cancer cells, so he insisted on removing the entire specimen intact (en bloc). In 1907 he reported in the medical literature his experience with 232 patients.[6]

Dr Halstead found that breast cancers in his patients were often large and bulky and sometimes hidden for years before the patient finally came to surgery. Some of those cancers involved deep penetration into the muscle. Others broke onto the chest wall disrupting the skin. Although these were far advanced neglected cases, Halstead reported that 32.2 percent survived 3 years and 29.8 percent lived 5 years or more.[6] These figures of late stage cancer survival compare very well with our results today. Although this was a disfiguring operation it was argued that the cure rate was better than any other procedure available. With improvement of surgical technique and control of infection, survival continued to improve until the 1940's and early 1950's. But from 1950 onward, the cure rate has not substantially improved. The surgery offered today is much less disfiguring, but is no better in effecting a cure than the Halstead operation of 1894.

The Halstead radical mastectomy was the standard battle plan that American surgeons depended upon, and all other procedures and treatments introduced since 1894 have invariably been compared to this surgical milestone.

Radical mastectomy was found to be fraught with morbidity and complications. Massive swelling of the arm was often encountered when lymphatic vessels and blood vessels were necessarily interrupted. Occasionally infection and nerve injuries were encountered. Stiffness and pain of the shoulder and scaring reeked havoc with rehabilitation efforts.

In view of these complications and the static cure rate over the past three generations, physicians and patients were soon looking for a new battle plan. In the mid-1950's clinicians in Europe and the United States were testing less radical alternatives for dealing with breast cancer. In England and France radiation therapy following limited surgery replaced the standard radical mastectomy as the bulwark of breast cancer control. Their results were good, although not quite as good as the Halstead procedure if cancer had already spread to the regional lymph nodes at the time of surgery or radiation treatment.

As later work would show, the dose of radiation used in those early European trials was insufficient. With an adjustment of the radiation it was shown that limited surgery with radiation was as good as the Halstead and with less complications. In 1975 Dr. Bernard Pierquin of Paris reported his 15 years experience using radiation following local excision of the tumor to control breast cancer.[7] The results were comparable to radical surgery.

In the 1960's American surgeons such as Dr John Madden in New York, and Dr George Crile, Jr, in Cleveland were openly critical of the Halstead operation for being too extensive.**8,9** Dr Crile became a vigorous advocate of less surgery; and in fact he lead the drive for the limited breast procedures performed today.

Meanwhile investigators in Europe including Dr. Handley of Middlesex Hospital, London, were challenging the sacred cow of radical mastectomy.**10** Data was presented advocating the modified radical mastectomy, a less disfiguring operation with comparable cure rates in early cancers. A new battle plan was in the making. Local control of the cancer, it was argued, could be achieved by removing the cancerous breast and contents of the axilla without compromising survival. Meyer and colleagues in Rockford, Illinois suggested in 1959 and again in 1978 that lesser procedures would have the same cure rate at ten years as the standard Halstead surgical procedure.**11** Then Dr Bernard Fisher, at the University of Pittsburgh, corroborated this finding in the national task force study of alternative breast cancer treatments.**12**

However, other breast specialists in America led by Anglem of Boston and Haagenson of New York, were not persuaded and continued to champion the cause of Halstead's radical approach. They pointed to the so-called Rotter lymph nodes found between the pectoralis major and minor muscles, that would be left behind unless the radical surgery was performed. In a blistering rebuttal to Dr Crile as late as 1974, Dr Anglem defended the radical mastectomy in the strongest terms and emotionally denigrated any lesser procedure.**13** He believed that Crile's data was biased. Anglem was joined by Dr Leis of New York, another Halstead devotee, in noting the high incidence of bilateral disease in young patients. He suggested prophylactic removal of the opposite breast in young cancer patients, in selected cases. Haagenson, a respected surgeon and pathologist at Columbia University, considered the modified radical mastectomy as a 'great leap backward'.**14,15**

About the same time, Dr Jerome Urban also of New York, was speaking at surgical gatherings around the country, advocating the radical Halstead and also the super-radical mastectomy if the lesion was located in the medial half of the breast.**16** He had reported his work in 1952 but had few supporters at that time. The super-radical in addition to the standard radical, consisted of removing the medial second, third and fourth ribs, along with the underlying lymph nodes. Urban claimed little increase in operating time and no significant morbidity. His statistics indicated an increased local recurrence if the super-radical was not done for cancer located in the medial half of the breast; however he could not claim increased survival at five and ten years. Very few surgeons followed his lead; and apparently no one could duplicate his results. The super-radical was out of step with the times.

American women were, by this time, demanding a more conservative approach and a greater voice in determining their treatment. Several investigators had shown that survival was not dependent on the location of the lesion in the breast. With increasing knowledge of the biology of the disease and improved weapons of chemotherapy, hormone therapy, and radiation, there was no longer any need to continue debating the utility of the super-radical procedure, or even, for that matter, the Halstead radical mastectomy.

THE MODIFIED RADICAL MASTECTOMY

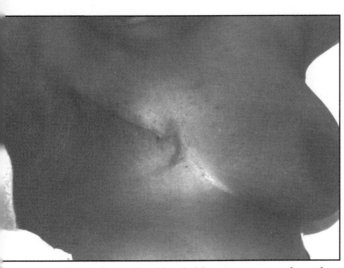

Fig. 9-1. Modified Radical Mastectomy is the standard surgery for breast cancer in the USA. This patient is ten years post-operative and doing well.

The most frequent operation for breast cancer performed today in the United States is the modified radical mastectomy or so-called "total mastectomy with axillary dissection." In this operation the cancerous breast is entirely removed including the nipple and a limited amount of skin. The muscles under the breast are preserved. The axillary contents are removed en bloc along with the breast.

Dr Donald Patey,

reporting in the British Journal of Cancer in 1967, described 156 cases operated in this manner between 1930 and 1943. **17** He removed the pectoralis minor muscle and spared the large pectoralis major. This has been modified; today both muscles are left in place. Patey used the term, "total mastectomy with axillary dissection". The results were good and comparable to the radical mastectomy, but there was little response in those years from surgeons on this side of the Atlantic. Neither Patey nor Handley of London was a match for Halstead's disciples. I suppose American surgeons were a bit provincial and favored the American way of doing things. The British surgeons did not claim that their operation held out any improvement in cure rate, only that it was less disfiguring. In the pre-1960's disfigurement was not of major concern to the American surgeons. The destruction of cancer was the only goal.

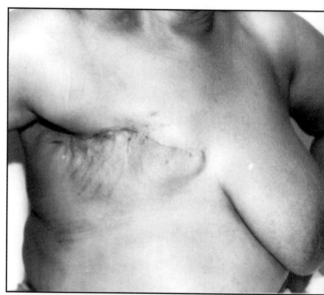

Fig. 9-2. **Modified Radical Mastectomy i many instances can be omitted in favor c lumpectomy, followed by radiation an chemotherapy. Several opinions should b sought before deciding on surgery. Plasti reconstruction following mastectomy ma be performed immediately after mastectom as part of the same operation.**

Over the ensuing 20 years a growing number of American doctors began to boldly support the notion of less surgery in early cases and avoiding mutilation without compromising the chance of cure. No doubt American medicine was responding to an outcry against too many tonsillectomies, too many hysterectomies and breast surgery that was too radical.

In the early 1970's Dr Delarue of Toronto General Hospital, found that modified radical mastectomy resulted in a comparable number of cures as the standard Halstead radical surgery, provided the muscle was not invaded and the apical nodes not involved.[18]

In 1977 Dr Bernard Fisher, in Pittsburgh, made his first report of clinical trials comparing radical mastectomy to total mastectomy with radiation.[19] After exhaustive analysis of the data, Dr Fisher and his colleagues concluded that there was no real difference with regards to survival between radical and modified radical surgery plus radiation. This proved true in early and advanced cancers.

In Dr Fisher's second report a look at the ten year results were available.[20] Again the data continued to support the notion that the radical mastectomy was not required in Stage I and Stage II disease when the muscle was not grossly involved. Many others have found no difference in long term survivorship between radical and modified radical surgery, coupled with radiation and chemotherapy.

PARTIAL MASTECTOMY

This surgical procedure championed by Crile and others since 1955 consists of excising a section of breast with the tumor along with the lower group of axillary nodes. The cure rate *overall* is not as good as the Halstead. In selected cases, however, according to Crile, the results are indeed comparable to radical surgery, and the contour of the breast is preserved. This means the lesion must be small and located in an outer quadrant and not fixed to the skin or underlying muscle. Few black patients present with these early lesions. Hence, few black women are amenable to this ultra-limited surgery.

If the cancer was small, localized to an outer quadrant, and the patient was relatively young with no other medical problems, Crile found that this limited surgery was every bit as curative as the Halstead radical surgery. Dr Crile reported 57 patients treated between 1955 and 1964 with a 67 percent five year overall control. Later results improved when this limited surgery was combined with radiation.[21] See *"Lumpectomy with Radiation"* later in this chapter.

Dr Umberto Veronesi of Milan, Italy, reported his experience using a quadrectomy (removal of the quadrant of breast bearing the cancer) with axillary dissection and radiation.22 His data over a fifteen year period was equal to the Halstead radical surgery without the mutilation, thus corroborating the work of Crile and others.

BILATERAL TOTAL MASTECTOMY

Removal of both breasts may seem justified in some women who are fearful of developing breast cancer when it is known that they carry the mutated breast cancer gene, BRCA1. Because of an 80 percent risk of contracting breast cancer before age 65, some women reason, and their surgeons may concur, that prophylactic removal of the breast would prevent a near certain development of cancer. See Chapter 5.

Prophylactic mastectomy may be done by making an incision in the crease just under the breast and raising a flap, excising the breast tissue and leaving the nipple intact. This method leaves a good deal of mammary tissue attached to the nipple area, and there are reports of cancer developing in this residual breast tissue.45

On the other hand when skin and nipple are removed along with the underlying breast, very little breast tissue is retained and the chance of cancer developing is diminished. In spite of exacting extirpation, any residual microscopic breast tissue left behind may theoretically serve as the nidus of cancer development. The protection of bilateral mastectomy from metastatic disease far outweighs the threat of cancer forming in any residual breast tissue left behind.44

This elective procedure must be approached with some trepidation. About half of the women who choose removal of both breasts have anxiety, depression, and personality change. About a third will have moderate to severe sexual problems after surgery. Careful screening may help identify women that may have fragile psychological underpinnings that may signal a potential psycho-social catastrophe.

In my opinion, careful surveillance every six months with the ever-improving mammography, the SPECT tomography, and the RODEO MRI, would be preferable to the prophylactic mastectomy and the emotional upheaval. See Chapter 3. I suspect the promise of gene therapy in the next ten years will replace the concept of bilateral mastectomy to lower the risk of breast cancer development in women with a genetic predisposition..

LUMPECTOMY WITH RADIATION

Since the early 1960's doctors in England and France have used excision of the cancer with only a small rim of normal tissue combined with radiation as their primary weapon. In over 95 percent of the cases the contour of the breast is preserved and they believe that their cure rate is as good as the radical Halstead. There is no serious doubt that radiation in adequate dose is able to kill micro-foci of breast cancer cells.

Radiation following lumpectomy is essential since it is known that most cancers are multi-centric in origin. In short, the major lump may be removed but residual microscopic tumor may be left in the remaining breast. A study at Memorial Hospital in New York showed that microscopic cancers that were unsuspected were found distant from the cancer lump in 26 percent of cases. It is not certain that these microscopic foci of cancer will ever become clinically important. In a study of women over seventy who died of causes other than breast cancer, microscopic cancer of the breast was found at a rate nineteen times expected for that age group. Microscopic thyroid cancers are also noted that never cause clinical cancer disease; and 40percent of elderly men have microscopic prostatic cancer that never becomes manifest.

Conservative surgery with radiation and even radiation alone in small cancers is widely available. Several States, including Massachusetts, California and Wisconsin have mandated that physicians inform patients with breast cancer of alternative treatments. See Appendix C. Clinical trials using radiation and limited, breast-saving surgery have been concluded by Dr Bernard Fisher; and the results in 1985 indicate that in early breast cancers limited surgery sparing the breast with post-operative radiation added can be as curative as more extensive surgery.23

The protocol usually is: The tumor is excised through a small incision and through a separate incision the lower lymph nodes from the axilla are removed. If there is cancer in those lymph nodes and the patient has not gone through menopause, she is also given chemotherapy, and in some cases, the anti-estrogen, Tamoxifen. Next, external beam orthovoltage, using either cobalt or the linear accelerator, is directed over the entire breast to remove any micro-foci of cancer. If the primary cancer is over 2.5 centimeters, Irridium can be implanted at the operative site to boost the radiation dose. External beam radiation is also directed over regional lymph nodes in the axillary, supraclavicular and internal mammary sites as well. A total of 5000 rads per week for 5 weeks controls microscopic invasive cancer in over 90 percent of cases. If axillary nodes are clinically enlarged, the dosage is boosted by 1000 to 2000 rads in that particular area.

In 1977 several medical centers in the U.S. reported results of a combined trial using radiation and local excision. The breast was spared and 75 percent of the patients had an excellent cosmetic result. Moreover they showed a five year survival of 91 percent in Stage I and 75 percent survival in Stage II patients. These figures compare very well with patients undergoing radical mastectomy.24 In 1982 the French provided proof that at 15 years the survival of patients with the lesser procedure and radiation were as good as the radical mastectomy.

At the Joint Center for Radiation Therapy, a prestigious cancer treatment center in Boston, Dr Martin Levene and others are treating breast cancer by local excision of the tumor, leaving the remainder of the breast intact, followed by local and regional radiation.25 Radiation is administered by external beam to the axilla, and Irridium is implanted at the site of the tumor excision if total removal is in doubt. In Stage I they report a 91 percent disease-free state at 5 years, and for Stage II a 60 percent disease-free state. Even Stage III showed a 26 percent survival at 5 years.

Some radiotherapists will accept only Stage I or Stage II women that are highly motivated to forego mastectomy. Some women faced with cancer continue to find greater security with mastectomy than radiation treatment; and there are surgeons who will not suggest to their patients a lumpectomy over a mastectomy even though it is available for those meeting certain criteria. It's the responsibility of the patients to question their doctors whether or not their case falls within the guidelines for lumpectomy and radiation.

Complications associated with radiation must be carefully considered. The patient routinely will find skin irritation, difficulty in swallowing and tracheitis (inflammation of the windpipe), esophagitis, and rarely rib fracture.

The immune system may be impaired, thus making the patient more susceptible to pneumonia and other infection. Serious complications, however, are unusual and should not dissuade the patient or the attentive radiotherapist. In a report from Harvard, 88 percent of a group of patients treated with radiation and followed up to seven years judged the cosmetic result as excellent or good.26 The texture of the breast may show increased firmness, and there may be a slight decrease in breast size. Often it is difficult to tell on casual inspection which breast was treated.

Despite occasional setbacks the trend towards a more prominent role for radiation and conservative surgery has altered the battle plan in the breast cancer war. In Stages I and II, the radical Halstead is a thing of the past. Only in Stage III with bulky tumors, with fixation against the chest wall would some surgeons perform a radical mastectomy. Dr Guy Robbins, former chief of the Breast Services of Memorial Hospital, New York, and other prominent surgeons, believed this was an indication for the Halstead radical mastectomy. On the other hand, Crile and Fisher, equally astute, declared that there was no place for radical breast surgery even in Stage III cancer; and indeed, the data seem to support their view.

The Blue Shield Plan of New Jersey reported that medical claims for radical mastectomy dropped 75 percent between 1974 and 1982 and the modified radical increased by 50 percent. All forms of breast amputation have continued to decrease in spite of the increased incidence of breast cancer. In the 1990's radical mastectomy is rarely done and any such procedure draws the immediate attention of peer review.

In 1995, through the work of Dr Bernard Fisher, the value of lumpectomy followed by radiation has been clearly delineated. Even after eliminating the erroneous records from a participating medical center (St Luc Hospital, Montreal, Canada), the data revealed that overall survival with lumpectomy and removal of lymph nodes with or without irradiation was equal to the modified radical mastectomy. With irradiation, however, recurrence in the affected breast was 10 percent compared to 35 percent without irradiation. However, the overall survival was *not* enhanced.38

LIMITED AXILLARY LYMPH NODE (SENTINEL) RESECTION

The first lymph node in the axilla that receives the first lymph flow from the breast is called the "sentinel node." It has been shown that if no cancer is present in this node, it is extremely unlikely that any other nodes will be positive for cancer. If the sentinel node could be examined, further extensive disection could be avoided if no cancer was found. This would eliminate further surgery in the axilla and eliminate most of the complications associated with removal of a large amount of tissue from the axilla, such as arm swelling and nerve damage. It also adds to the accuracy of cancer staging and prognostic conclusions.[55,56]

SURGERY AND THE MENSTRUAL CYCLE

Did you know that breast cancer survival is related to when definitive surgery is performed with respect to the menstrual period? The prognosis is considerably enhanced when mastectomy or other surgery is performed during the latter half of the cycle, about ten days before menstruation is due. Studies have shown that when examining a large group of women with all stages of disease, a ten year survival in the first group was 72 percent compared to 40 percent survival for those operated before day 12 of the menstrual cycle (p=.001). The first 12 days of the cycle, called the follicular phase is characterized by surging blood levels of estrogen. See Chapter 2. The next 12-16 days, called the luteal phase, reflects falling estrogen in preparation for the menstrual flow.[43]

AFTER SURGERY WHAT COMES NEXT—RADIATION OR CHEMOTHERAPY?

As late as 1996 the optimal sequencing of chemotherapy and radiation following lumpectomy was in dispute. Until the 1980's surgeons agreed that radiation followed surgery and then hormones, chemotherapy and whatever else was out there came last.

However, with the growing popularity of limited surgery, the use of

Tamoxifen, and a better understanding of the role of chemotherapy, choices of treatment are no longer that simple. Investigators demonstrated that chemotherapy given first held an advantage if it was suspected that distant spread had already taken place. There was also some discussion as to when the chemotherapy should begin following surgery—within hours or days or after several weeks. There seems to be no advantage in starting chemotherapy immediately or waiting several weeks.**31**

If there are three or more positive cancer nodes in the axilla at the time of surgery, distal metastasis is very likely and early systemic chemotherapy would be in order followed later by radiation therapy for local control. However if surgery reveals no nodes or only one or two in the axilla and examination of the excised breast cancer suggests that some margins were not removed with the specimen, then local control with radiation should occur first with chemotherapy to follow.

Harvard researchers addressed this question and reported their findings in 1996. They concluded that if there is a high risk of metastasis, a 12 week course of chemotherapy should begin after surgery, and then followed by standard radiation therapy. It was noted that at 5 years distal metastasis was 36 percent in the radiation first group compared to 25 percent in the chemotherapy first cohort. This difference was statistically significant ($p=0.05$). The overall survival was 81 percent in the chemotherapy first group compared to 73 percent in the radiation first group ($p=0.11$).**30**

HORMONES AND CHEMOTHERAPY

As new potent weapons are developed, strategy and tactics will obviously change. We now find in our arsenal a growing array of drugs and hormones. These armaments are now ready and available to assail the metastatic cancer that is often in transit when the gross breast cancer is first discovered. Consequently, many clinicians believe that all Stage III women should have chemotherapy, and Stage II patients as well. Preliminary reports are suggesting that the outlook was improved, and perhaps one can be cured by adding chemotherapy immediately at the time of limited surgery. This data has been developed by Fisher, and if it can be duplicated and corroborated, it will represent a major assault on the barricades of breast cancer.27

From 1945 to 1960 hormone therapy (estrogen, testosterone, and castration) was the major weapon in the control of metastatic breast cancer. But the physician had no way to predict the response and it was actually a shot in the dark proposition. A few of the patients that did have a remission could expect additional control with removal of the adrenal glands or hypophysectomy. However the morbidity and mortality of these operations was formidable.

Between 1960 and 1970 single agent chemotherapy was in vogue, almost completely replacing hormone treatment. These weapons led to excess morbidity and mortality as dosage requirements and tolerance of the patient were not completely elucidated.

The years 1970 to 1975 saw the emergence of combination chemotherapy (the use of more than one anti-cancer drug) with improved longevity. The combination most often used in the U.S. then and now include CMF (cyclophosphamide, methyltrexate, 5-florouracil), and CAF (cyclophosphamide, Adriamycin, 5-florouracil) for advanced cancer. L-pam (l-phenylalanine mustard) plus 5-florouracil found some success in Stage II premenopausal patients at the time of limited surgery.

In 1993, CMF continued to be the standard chemotherapy for breast cancer. The drugs are combined with Tamoxifen in all Stage II patients of all ages that are estrogen receptor (ER) positive. By 1996 general guide-lines governing the use and expected response to chemotherapy continued to be refined and were made available to all breast cancer patients.

The most important predictors of recurrence is the size of the cancer and the number of cancer positive lymph nodes in the axilla found at the time of surgery. Without chemothcrapy, 1-3 nodes gives a 45-60 percent recurrence rate, 4-9 nodes causes a 50-75 percent recurrence, and 10 or more nodes will lead to recurrence in 90 percent of cases. If there are no positive nodes, the recurrence may vary from 5-50 percent in ten years. In this case the size of the cancer is more of a determinant factor. For example, if the original cancer is less than 1 centimeter in greatest diameter, the recurrence rate is 5-10 percent at ten years. If the tumor is over 2 centimeters, the recurrence rate is 20 percent at ten years. A third predictor is the presence of cancer cells in the lymph channels and capillaries immediately adjacent to the cancer.**39**

In women under age 35 and in black women metastasis and mortality may be somewhat higher due to a faster cancer cell growth rate in these women.**40**

The next obvious question is, "How much improvement in survival can we expect when adjuvant chemotherapy and Tamoxifen are added to the local control by surgery and radiation?" The answer is found in pooling the medical literature and examining the consensus data. Chemotherapy has its greatest response in women under age 50. On the other hand Tamoxifen has a greater benefit in older post-menopausal women. If a cancer is estrogen receptor positive, there is a small additional benefit of Tamoxifen use in younger women.

A patient may gain some idea of what benefit chemotherapy will afford by multiplying risk of recurrence according to tumor size by recurrence according to lymph node status.

TAMOXIFEN

Since 1976, a new battery of cancer-fighting tools called antiestrogens have been brought to the struggle. The most common agent in this class is Tamoxifen. By 1992 it had been fairly well tested by Dr Fisher and his colleagues and a definite place in the treatment protocol was outlined.**29** By 1995 Tamoxifen became the most widely prescribed medication to combat breast cancer. It was noted to reduce breast cancer recurrence in the opposite breast of cancer patients by 40 percent. It is now being tested to determine if it is useful in normal women to prevent de nouveau occurrence of breast cancer. Final results of this study should be available by the year 2010.

Essentially Tamoxifen blocks the action of estrogen which is thought to perpetuate cancer. If a breast cancer patient has a high level of estrogen receptor (ER) positive cells, she will almost always respond to Tamoxifen. On the other hand, women who are ER negative or have a low positive rate, respond less, if at all, to Tamoxifen.

The side effects of Tamoxifen in young women are a sudden

menopause. In fact hot flashes, night sweats and personality changes may preclude the use of Tamoxifen in some women. There is a slight risk of inducing uterine cancer, but benefit far outweighs the risk. Tamoxifen lowers cholesterol and lowers the risk of osteoporosis and coronary heart disease. The drug should not be taken with birth control pills; nor should it be taken during pregnancy. The National Cancer Institute suggests taking the drug for five years, since there seems to be no greater benefit in women who have taken the drug for longer periods.[32]

Tamoxifen can be combined with standard chemotherapy and it has been shown to give added benefit especially in those patients over 50 years of age. This antiestrogen is being used more and more in cases that formerly were treated with hypophysectomy or adrenalectomy.

Other antiestrogens are currently undergoing trials. **Megestrol** is being used in women who are resistant to Tamoxifen. An investigational antiestrogen called **ICI 182780** appears to double the remission of Tamoxifen when compared to Megestrol. ICI 182780 has shown no side effects except a burning pain at the injection site in 10 percent of patients. An oral form is being developed. It does not cause menopausal symptoms such as hot flashes and perspiration as in some cases of Tamoxifen users. ICI 182780 is less likely to cause uterine cancer and protects against osteoporosis better than Tamoxifen.

The Vitamin A derivative, **4-HPR**, has shown positive results in preventing recurrence of breast cancer in the remaining breast in premenopausal patients.[49]

Toremifene, another antiestrogen drug works in the same manner as Tamoxifen, with equal efficacy. Side effects appear to be less and cholesterol lowering effects are more impressive.

The first example of a new class of drugs called "Selective Estrogen Receptor Modulators (SERMS) is **Raloxifene**. This drug works much like Tamoxifen in that it has been proven in laboratory animals to sgnificantly prevent breast cancer. It appears to have fewer side effects and does not cause uterine cancer. Trials will soon be underway comparing Raloxifene and Tamoxifen with regards efficacy and side-effects. Currently Raloxifene is FDA approved to prevent osteoporosis.

RU-486

RU-486 was in the news some years ago when it was introduced to the United States as an abortion pill, obviating the need for the usual surgical method of abortion. However, mifepristone (RU-486) has also been studied as a therapy in advanced breast cancer.

While Tamoxifen blocks the effects of estrogen, mifepristone (RU-486) and onapristone combat breast cancer by interfering with progesterone and thus inhibiting the growth of some breast cancers that depend on progesterone along with estrogen. In laboratory animals RU-486 has shown clearly that it does indeed fight breast cancer; and when used along with Tamoxifen, the drugs are synergetic and complement one another, blocking both estrogen and progesterone.

Clinical trials in France and Canada are on-going to determine the role of antiprogestin medications and how they might augment the treatment with Tamoxifen. See Appendix D regarding breast cancer clinical trials in the United States.

TAXOL

Taxol (paclitaxel) is an investigational drug that has limited usefulness in about 30 percent of advanced ovarian cancer cases. Although it was found to have anti-cancer activity by the National Cancer Institute in the 1960's, it was not until 1989 that researchers at the Johns Hopkins University demonstrated shrinkage or complete disappearance in 30 percent of women with advanced ovarian cancer. In 1992 Taxol was approved by the FDA for treatment of resistant ovarian cancers.

Since that time, Taxol has shown promise in the treatment of advanced breast cancers along with other major cancers. Trials are being conducted even as I write.

Paclitaxel is derived from the bark of the Pacific yew tree. The extraction and manufacture is complex and it requires an enormous amount of the raw product to produce the drug. Hence the ongoing trials are hampered by the limited supply. Great efforts are underway to find alternative sources in related plants and trees as well as developing a laboratory source of the active ingredient. Since 1989 Bristol-Myers Squibb, a leading drug company, has been supplying formulated paclitaxel under the proprietary name Taxol.

The French have recently developed a Taxol analogue, that is, a drug related to Taxol, with similar anticancer properties. It is called Taxotere. They have agreed to allow the NCI to use this drug in clinical trials.

Within the next few years it is expected that Taxotere will gain complete FDA approval for treatment of advanced breast cancer.**41** Currently this drug can only be used in clinical trials. To enter a clinical trial one should contact the National Cancer Institute at 1 800 4 CANCER.

IMMUNOTHERAPY

The immune system is that set of mechanisms incorporated in the body to help defend itself against invading bacteria, viruses, foreign matter, and cancer. One gains immunity when the body recognizes a particle, a substance, or a cancer as a foreign intruder. The intruder is called an antigen. The body, through an elaborate system in response to the antigen, produces antibodies designed to resist and destroy the invader. The antibody is sometimes very specific and will attack only the antigen that caused the specific antibody to form.

Other antibodies are not specific and will go about destroying all foreign substances. For example, it has been found that the bacterium C. parvum will stimulate the production of antibodies against not only this particular antigen but also against certain cancer cells as well. It has been shown that patients receiving chemotherapy survive much longer when this antigen, C. parvum, is incorporated in the protocol.

In another example, it is known that Bacillus Calumette Guerre (BCG) serves as an antigen against Mycobacteria bovis. It stimulates antibody formation not only against M. bovis but also against M. tuberculosis, thus immunizing against tuberculosis. For some unknown reason it also can offer some protection against certain cancers. In Stage II, breast cancer investigators using BCG noted only a 5 percent relapse rate compared to a 40 percent relapse rate in patients not using BCG. Levamisole, another antigen, with non-specificity in antibody formation is also being tried in the search for cancer immunotherapy.

In spite of the appeal of immunotherapy the results have not been consistent. There's still too many unanswered questions, and overall, it has not been a reliable weapon in treating early or late stages of breast cancer. Consequently, immunotherapy, that is, using the immune system to control cancer, remains experimental and only controlled trials are being conducted. It is not available for most patients. Several protocols combining immunotherapy with chemotherapy, radiation and/or surgery are being suggested. It remains to be seen whether or not a protocol of hormones and immunotherapy combined will find a place in preventive or palliative care. This points up the need for clinical trials. See Chapter 7.

In 1994, Dr H K Lyerly, and his colleagues at Duke University, began trials of immune therapy on women with Stage IV breast cancer. It had been shown in mice that breast cancer cells, genetically altered and then implanted back into mice with breast cancer, would stimulate killer cells that would attack and kill the cancer.

Dr Lyerly proposed to inject each woman with her own malignant cells that had been altered. When injected, cytokine interleukin-2 is formed that has the ability to kill breast cancer tissue. If this approach is successful, it will become a major weapon in destroying metastatic breast cancer. The project was approved by the National Cancer Institute and the FDA.33

MEDICATIONS ON THE HORIZON

Endostatin and **Angiostatin** are two of the most prominent drugs under study that inhibit the development of blood vessels that are necessary for the growth of cancers. Cancers simply can not grow if their blood supply is denied. Judah Folkman, MD at the Children's Hospital in Boston has shown excellent prevention of cancer growth using these drugs in laboratory animals. These drugs effectively reduce the bulk of cancer and allow standard chemotherapy to to be more effective. It is also believed that these drugs may encourage cancer dormancy even after chemotherapy is no longer effective. I expect trials and approval of this approach by the year 2000. **Marimastat** and **Thalidomide**, that inhibit cancer growth by interfering with blood vessel formation are also being tested in breast cancer as well as in prostate and other cancers.

Herceptin (Trastuzumab) was developed to specifically attack cancers that harbor the over-expressed gene HER2/neu. Ordinary cells carry two copies of this gene and several receptor sites on the cell surface. In 30 percent of breast cancer patients, the cancer cells carry many many copies of the gene HER2/neu and hundreds of receptor sites. The receptor sites are the point of attachment of cancer cells that harbor the HER2/neu gene. This is how the cancer cells grow, by attaching to each other athe receptor site. The Herceptin drug is a monoclonal antibody, or a mirror of the HER2/neu, and as such can attach to the receptor site, blocking a cancer cell with the true HER2/neu from attaching to that site. If the cancer cells can not attach to each other, their growth is stopped. Indeed cancer have been shrunk to microscopic size using Herceptin for many months. It is being tried with chemotherapy and other treatments. The final answer is not in, but the direction is promising.

BONE MARROW TRANSPLANTS

The problem with chemotherapy is that as it kills the cancer cells it also kills the bone marrow essential for life. Therefore the dosage of chemotherapy is limited. In the 1980's it sounded like a good idea to first remove bone marrow and then give highly concentrated chemotherapy to kill cancer cells. Bone marrow could then be replaced after treatment and the patient would benefit and not be harmed at the same time. The procedure is called autologous bone marrow transplant (ABMT). The term 'autologous' means that marrow taken from the patient, will be returned to the same patient at a later time.

In 1990 the first NCI approved trial was underway. But recruiting women to enter the trials has been sluggish. There has been so much hype in the press lauding the value of ABMT that women do not want to be randomized into a group that will not get the bone marrow treatment.

The trials are so far behind schedule due to lack of patients willing to participate that it will be well into the next century before we know whether or not bone marrow transplants are actually worthwhile. Only one of the twelve major medical insurers require that patients be part of a clinical trial to receive payment for the procedure. The rest of the insurance companies rather pay the $80,000 to $150,000 price per treatment, simply to avoid public pressure and potential lawsuits.

Our current knowledge indicates that the procedure has no particular advantage over standard multi-drug chemotherapy, which cost $15,000 to $40,000. Nonetheless the procedure continues to grow in popularity. There were only 522 treatments in 1989 compared to over 4000 in 1994 according to the United States General Accounting Office.

THE BATTLE PLAN TODAY

In reviewing the overall strategy developed since 1970, our first line of defense and our most potent weapon remains surgery. Either the modified radical mastectomy, or lumpectomy plus radiation with separate removal of axillary nodes for Stages I and II, would be appropriate.

The Halstead radical mastectomy for Stage III cancer is rarely advocated in most major centers; and most surgeons, I suspect, will not find the need for radical surgery in any circumstance. Preoperative radiation and chemotherapy are useful to shrink the large cancers to allow modified radical mastectomy.

If there is local spread to lymph nodes as in Stage II then chemotherapy and Tamoxifen would be in order in the estrogen-receptor positive pre-menopausal patient. Some doctors would use these agents prophylactically even if there are no obvious metastases. In the estrogen negative patient, Tamoxifen will be much less effective.

In the post-menopausal patient, under similar conditions, similar surgery and radiation, followed by Tamoxifen is the standard care today for the estrogen receptor positive patient. Chemotherapy is usually withheld in estrogen negative patients unless there is clear evidence of metastasis. This is because the side effects of chemotherapy can not be justified in the face of the known poor therapeutic results of chemotherapy in older women.

The combination of chemotherapy, Tamoxifen,and palliative radiotherapy is usually prescribed in Stage IV breast cancer.

There continues to be lingering skepticism with regards sparing the breast and combining very limited surgery with radiation or chemotherapy. The data seem impressive. I expect the use of limited surgery, followed by chemotherapy and radiation will continue to increase in the United States and eventually become the treatment of choice in this country as it is in Europe.

Some physicians prefer chemotherapy over radiation because radiation only kills the local cancer. Chemotherapy at the time of limited surgery kills not only local cancer but metastatic foci as well. There is mounting evidence in pre-menopausal women that early chemotherapy at the time of surgery is beneficial.

The second line of defense becomes a holding action. This applies to patients who've had a relapse following initial control of their disease. In this phase we are concerned with prolonging life, easing pain, and enhancing the quality of life. The weapons used depend on the estrogen-receptor (ER) status of the cancer. If it is positive then a majority of post-menopausal patients will respond to Tamoxifen. For the ER negative patients and most pre-menopausal women we must retreat immediately to chemotherapy.

The ER positive women who respond to removal of the ovaries will often have a second remission following adrenalectomy or hypophysectomy. However, because of attendant morbidity and complications this drastic surgery is no longer in vogue. Tamoxifen, the anti-estrogen that has been effective in post-menopausal women, has replaced radical intervention.

The majority of women with Stage I or II are cured today with the weapons we have at hand, but the ultimate victory in more advanced cases may require more sophisticated intervention. In the coming decades, artillery now on the drawing boards will be added to the battle plan. New combinations of surgery, chemotherapy, radiotherapy, hormonal therapy, immunotherapy and gene therapy may well be part of tomorrow's arsenal to combat cancer. Even hyperthermia (heating the cancer or the whole body) associated with radiation has shown promise in better controlling breast cancer in a series of clinical Phase III trials.[54]

Interferon, a substance produced by the body in response to viral invasion and other attacks, appears to enhance the immune system. It also appears to stimulate anti-tumor killer cells to destroy cancer. In one study 25 percent of patients with advanced breast cancer found remission with Interferon treatment. However, there have been unacceptable side effects, and supply and purity have also been a problem.

It has been found that cancer cells require cysteine to proliferate, invade, and spread. In the laboratory animal if this essential amino acid is removed from the body, cancer cells die; however, before it proves fatal to the animal, cysteine can be replaced. Cysteine testing is now in Phase I trials.[47] There are many other substances also undergoing testing to determine their potency in thwarting the breast cancer enemy.[48] (Appendix D).

On the horizon is the possibility of gene therapy. In 1996, Dr Roy Jensen from Vanderbilt University reported preliminary work in which copies of the BRCA1 gene could be introduced into ovarian cancer patients to replace their own mutated (damaged) BRCA1 gene. The new gene it was theorized would then work as the damaged gene would have in suppressing ovarian cancer. This should also be workable for breast cancer. Phase I trials were started on patients with advanced ovarian cancer. By 2006 we should have information of the feasibility of gene therapy in ovarian and breast cancer. Obviously this would pose a major victory in the war on breast cancer.

THE BATTLE FOR FAIRNESS
IN THE CARE OF AFRICAN-AMERICAN WOMEN

Not only must black women and their doctors be aware of the dynamic battle plan in the war on breast cancer, but it is equally vital that they be ever vigilant regarding the potential and sometimes real discrepancies in the care provided black women vis-a-vis white women.[34,35,45] A study of United States hospitals revealed that on average, black patients receive fewer hospital services and are treated with less intensity than expected when matched against white patients with similar health characteristics.[42]

In a recent report it was noted that black women were referred less often for mammography. It is assumed that mammography decreases breast cancer mortality and frequency of obtaining mammography is based on the number of clinical encounters. It is also assumed that mortality in black women is higher than found in white women because the black women fail to get mammograms. However, in this study of 3,187,116 Medicare recipients in 10 States, it was found that when black and white women were divided into groups according to the number of medical office visits during the year, the more visits (1, 2, 3 visits) the more likely mammogram was performed. But at each level black women were referred less often than whites. For an example, in women who saw a doctor three times in a year the number of mammograms ordered was higher than in the group that visited a doctor two times a year. But when divided by race, regardless of the number of visits, black women always lagged behind their white counterparts.[50]

It was documented in 1986, that Medicaid women, disproportionately African-American, with breast cancer who underwent lumpectomy received post-operative radiation treatment 45 percent of the time compared to 78 percent of the time for private patients. By 1990 the figure increased to 60 percent for the Medicaid women.[52] Omission of radiation treatment directly affects the chance of recurrence.[51] Without radiation treatment, cancer returns in ten years in an additional 50 percent in those women who did not receive the post-operative radiotherapy.

Other investigators have found significant discrepancies in treatment protocols depending on socio-economic status.[53,54]

These examples represent simple proof that black women must speak up and demand not only regular screening mammography but standard care as well; and you and I must be their advocate.

Reports in the medical literature must be read with a keen eye when the author glosses over the poor survival of black women and intimates that it is somehow the fault of the victim and not inferior or sub-par treatment.

In a report comparing the treatment of Stage II breast cancer in black and white women, the authors concluded that blacks and whites received the same surgical care and post-operative chemotherapy and Tamoxifen. Upon a closer reading we find that the authors admit that blacks are generally relegated to mastectomy rather than lumpectomy. They try to attribute this to the large size of tumors in black women, but they fail to point out that even if the tumor is large in a white patient, lumpectomy is still done. Nor do they point out that even if the tumor is small in a black woman, mastectomy is done. The report states..."recommendations for treatment in blacks and whites were reviewed (data not shown).."

However, the article points out that under age 50, whites had standard chemotherapy in 54 percent of cases compared to 46 percent for blacks. For all age groups, 34 percent for whites and 27 percent for blacks received chemotherapy.

With regards combined chemotherapy and Tamoxifen, 17 percent of whites received the combination compared to 11 percent of black women.

Finally, 29 percent of whites received radiation treatment with or without chemotherapy and/or Tamoxifen, compared to 22 percent for blacks.**36** They do not deal with the report that radiation treatment combined with chemotherapy, may enhance a disease free state.**46** The upshot is that different conclusions can be drawn from the same medical report depending on one's point of view.

In another article investigators go to great length in contrasting black and white breast cancer patients with regards marital status, poverty index, education, medical insurance, and occupation. Pages are devoted to these details highlighting the blight of the black community which they also admit has little or nothing to do with breast cancer. They talk about the larger tumors and the more frequent metastasis in black women when first diagnosed. But nowhere does anyone suggest that for black women we must look for cancer earlier when the cancer is small and localized. How better can the mortality gap be closed?

In the same report it is stated, "Treatment data collected by this study were limited. Specific chemotherapeutic agents administered were recorded but the amount and schedule of chemotherapy was not collected..." In another paragraph they state, "....treatment information did not explain any of the survival difference between blacks and whites." How could it when complete treatment information was not included for the reader's examination? The article goes on to instruct, "Future efforts should emphasize community educational efforts...and increased compliance with current screening recommendations." In other words it is the victims' fault. And yet the investigators in the same report concede that black women with breast cancer are less likely to have a surgical procedure or radiation treatment. **37** Nor do they point out that even when black women follow current screening guidelines mortality is consistently higher than the mortality in white women.

Since there is so much difference between the races with regards incidence, response to treatment and the natural course of the disease, not to mention variance in care, we need trials based on parameters uniquely found in black women. See Chapters 7 and 9.

The breast cancer enemy is being challenged and confronted on the battlefield of science and technology. Breakthroughs in early diagnosis and treatment are in the offing. For the black community to properly benefit in this technological revolution, African-American women must mobilize for mutual support and dissemination of information to prepare themselves for personal participation in treatment and diagnostic decisions. Information is the first step to survival. The second step is application. The third step is vigilance.

———

For the past several years black women breast cancer survivors all over this country have begun to mobilize and network. They speak to the needs of their own like no one else can or will. In the next chapter we shall become acquainted with some of the Sisters who are taking steps to make a difference through organized effort and dedication.

CHAPTER TEN

ISTER TO SISTER
African American Women Networking

Support groups can, to some degree, alleviate the profound psychological depression that sometimes accompanies newly diagnosed breast cancer.[1,2] It is even more helpful when members of a support group are similar in race and culture and language. In the American Cancer Society's Reach to Recovery Program described in Chapter 12, this similarity is considered paramount when matching long-term survivors to newly treated breast cancer patients.

There is no doubt that when women get together to share coping strategies their lives are enhanced, their focus is sharpened, and their energies are combined and directed. There is some evidence that social ties and support networks increase longevity more so for black breast cancer survivors than their white counterparts.[4]

Breast cancer survivors networking with common purpose can only be a good thing. The definition of life and service become finely tuned. Worthy projects are identified. These women discover that a mind in action cannot dwell on the negative when there is good work to be done. A life with purpose will not be lived in vain.

There has been a proliferation of breast cancer survivor organizations since the early 1990's. These groups have emerged to empower women and to provide a clarion voice to speak to their demands and point of view.[3] For black women it was not long before they realized that their needs could not be adequately addressed by a Caucasian dominated organization. Certainly the guidance of the Susan G Komen Fund, the American Cancer Society, the National Breast Cancer Coalition, and other organizations were absolutely vital to survival and growth, but the coping strategies and nurturing at the local level had to come from the innate black cultural and social structure.

It may be the language, the music, the religion, the dress, the smell, the hair, the skin color, the laugh, or just the comfort level that the Sisters share—that go into the mix of making a group relative to the individual's needs. Black breast cancer survivors needed to be where their voices would be heard. Who wants to be simply tolerated and treated politely when breast cancer mortality is 16 percent higher, and there is bias in diagnosis and treatment for black women?

Black women are asking, "If we don't take responsibility for ourselves, who will?" They are beginning to understand that the 21st century will be a time dominated by a health maintenance-insurance industrial complex bent on cost containment and, let's face it, the rationing of health care. The system must be confronted and challenged. Black women and breast cancer survivors must pool their knowledge and coping methodologies to make the delivery of optimum health care real and accessible in their communities. The notion is simple but still rings true: "In Unity there is Strength."

Here are some examples of how African-American breast cancer survivors are coming together, to throw out the lifeline, so to speak, to save themselves and a community too often shoved aside and overlooked:

———

The Arkansas Witness Project

I was the guest author at an affair in Washington, DC, in 1994; and at that meeting I became acquainted with a group of black women from the Arkansas Witness Project. I was so impressed that I must tell you about it. The Witness Project is a group of black women who are breast cancer survivors. They range in age from young to old. Their motto is: "In church, people witness to save souls. At the Witness Project, we witness to save lives."

These breast cancer survivors comprise a health education program that speaks directly to the cultural needs of the black community. They take the message of breast cancer awareness to black churches on a regular basis, and present themselves as a living testament demonstrating that early

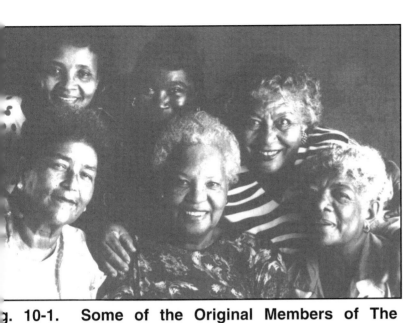

detection can save lives, and that life can be satisfying and fulfilling even after the cancer demon strikes. They encourage church members sitting in the pews to promise to get a mammogram on the very next opportunity. They even suggest how mammograms are

ɉ. 10-1. Some of the Original Members of The ʞansas Witness Project

available without charge for the needy.

In 1993, less than 15 percent of eligible African-American women got a mammogram. Compare that to 50 percent of eligible white women. These wonderful women from Little Rock have a big job on their hands; but it's something that should be duplicated all over the country.

Dr Deborah Erwin, PhD, and her associates at the University of Arkansas Medical Center (Arkansas Cancer Research Center), developed the idea of black women talking to black audiences about breast cancer several years ago. But it was more than just an idea. Dr Erwin, with dedication and hard work, made sure that the program got off the ground. She and her colleagues were instrumental in establishing the connections and getting the funding. Presently, the Witness Project is supported by the American Cancer Society, the Avon Breast Health Fund, the Susan G Komen Breast Cancer Fund, and other organizations with a national scope. They've produced a marvelous 20 minute video that I've used on occasion when talking to groups about breast cancer awareness. If you are contemplating forming a support group in your area, you may wish to contact the Arkansas Witness Project. They provide a loose-leaf instruction guide detailing how a program can be set up and administered. Suggestions for funding and community projects are also described.

I can't say enough about Dr Deborah Erwin. I saw her on C-SPAN back in 1993 at the Breast Cancer Conference, hosted by Secretary Donna Shalala. When Dr Erwin gave a short presentation about the Witness Project, it was obvious to me that here was a special person who was moving to make a difference.

The glaring mortality figures among black women could be overcome if there were more souls like Dr Erwin, who have the capacity to extend themselves beyond the esoteric to the practical, beyond the potential to the kinetic, beyond the doublespeak to the "for real."

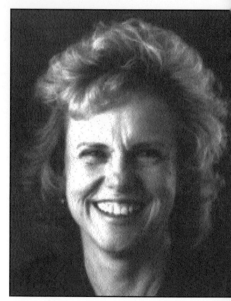

But Doctor Erwin couldn't have done it without those stalwart survivors who have each faced their own personal fear and tested their individual faith. It takes courage to stand up in front of strangers and

Fig. 10-2. Deborah Erwin, PhD

say, "I've lost a breast to cancer. I'm living day by day. As long as I'm able, whether it's ten days or ten years, I want to encourage you to face up to your responsibility for yourself, your family and your children. Get regular check-ups, do breast self examinations and get a mammogram on a regular basis. Breast cancer can be cured almost always if you catch it in time."

The black community owes much to these women, in Little Rock, for coming together for mutual support, and trust; and taking the responsibility to get the message out.

———

The Breast Cancer Resource Committee

In 1978 Belva Brown Brissett was diagnosed with breast cancer. In 1981 her sister, Zora Brown, was also diagnosed. Both received the standard treatment of the time but Belva had a recurrence and was treated a second and then a third time. By 1989 these two black women, realizing the disparity between the incidence, diagnosis, and mortality between black and white women, joined with several others to form the Breast Cancer Resource Committee.

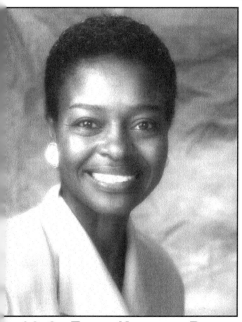

Since its founding, the organization has worked tirelessly to heighten awareness among African-American women of the dangers of breast cancer. Based in Washington, DC, this group has achieved a national reputation for their work in the black community. They have attracted recognition and funding from major contributors and leading advocacy groups such as the American Cancer Society and the Susan G Komen Fund.

Until her passing, Belva Brown Brissett worked shoulder to shoulder with her sister, Zora, in getting the message out: "Breast Cancer can be cured if detected early." They continued to hammer home the theme that black women were not being informed and were not being screened in satisfactory numbers. Today the Greater Southeast Healthcare System has established the Belva Brissett Advocacy Center.

Fig. 10-3. **Zora Kramer Brown**

This Center provides training and education to volunteers dedicated to disseminate information concerning breast cancer to black women, where they live and worship. Screening and education are the major goals.

Zora Kramer Brown, Belva's sister, has survived breast cancer more than 15 years. And she has used her time wisely. She did not bury her talent. She didn't shield her lamp under a bushel. Zora has worked diligently to make the Breast Cancer Resource Committee what it is today. Her good works glow from the hilltop of achievement. Her cheerful electric smile is truly caring, and real, and committed. She is a daily blessing to African-American women threatened by breast cancer.

Zora lives her life with a high calling. Not in step with the frivolity and nonsense of the now. But attuned to the drum beat of righteous concern about African-Americans and their lack of breast cancer awareness. Her life is dedicated to changing all that through coalition building and innovation.

To that end in 1993, Rise-Sister-Rise was organized as a breast cancer survivor support group, with an Afrocentric tilt. Rise-Sister-Rise has formed a nidus where women of color could come together and simply "let their hair down," be themselves, ask questions, exchange information, and just be with the sisters. A curriculum has been developed to cover breast cancer topics so that solid information can be imparted and passed on to other women.

For more information I invite you to get in touch with Zora Kramer Brown at the Breast Cancer Resource Committee at 202 463 8040.

———

The Sisters Network

On October 20, 1996, the Sisters Network in Houston, Texas, kicked off their third annual Gift For Life Block Walk, designed to target the black community with information about breast cancer and encourage periodic examinations to enhance the chance of cure. Over two hundred volunteers canvassed underserved Houston's Sunnyside neighborhood, disseminating 6000 educational pamphlets, taking the message directly to the people. This was not a political venture— "do this for me and I'll do that for you." No. This was "do this for yourself and your loved ones and everyone will benefit, especially you."

The Gift For Life Block Walk was a matter of good people coming together and pooling there intellect and talent. They recognized a need in the black community and were willing to step out on faith, and go where the people dwell to instruct and inform. Their target was a vulnerable black people who receive too little attention in spite of a breast cancer menace that disproportionately invades the African-American community. Organizing the event, procuring the literature and handouts, making the posters, alerting the media, and finding the volunteers, didn't just happen. It was caring black women, mostly breast cancer survivors, who made up the Sisters Network, who were willing to put in the time and effort to assure the success of the Gift For Life Block Walk. They were joined by nurses, social workers, cancer survivors, housewives, maids and simply a cross-section of the people they intended to alert.

Sisters Network is the first, and, as of 1997, the only, African-American Breast Cancer Survivors Support Group with a national scope , organized and governed by breast cancer survivors. They are dedicated to unconditional acceptance of all members, as they provide a sanctuary

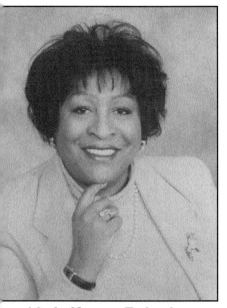

where the mind, body and spirit can be nurtured and celebrated. They believe that the holistic approach is one of the ways that human needs can be addressed. Their motto: "In Unity there is STRENGTH. In strength there is POWER. In power there is CHANGE."

The origins of Sisters Network go back to 1994, when Karen E Jackson, a breast cancer survivor, appreciated the need for black women survivors to come together for mutual support and exchange of information. She was able to direct her energies and focus her determination to provide the catalyst for an organization of black women that now numbers ten chapters (See Appendix B), and promises to continue multiplying across the nation.

g. 10-4. Karen E Jackson

Sisters Network has an ongoing agenda. These women are about networking on a national scale with the American Cancer Society, the National Breast Cancer Coalition, and the National Coalition for Cancer Survivorship (NCCS). They are about providing free mammograms, free prostheses, and providing speakers and outreach projects.

They are also about raising funds to target their agenda. In December, 1995, they had a successful fund raiser with the opening of the movie, "Waiting To Exhale" with Whitney Houston and Angela Bassett.

Their efforts were recognized by the NCCS in 1996. Sisters Network was awarded the Outstanding Program Award in Minority Cancer Survivorship. In 1997 Sisters Network National President, Karen E Jackson received the prestigious Hope Award [The Volunteer of the Year Award] at the 6th Biennial Symposium on Minorities, the Medically Underserved & Cancer.

Sisters Network publishes a Quarterly Newsletter, distributed nationally, that highlights their activities and provides useful information. If you would like to organize breast cancer survivors in your community and be affiliated with Sisters Network, contact Karen E Jackson at (713) 781-0255

———

SisterReach Advisory Council

Experience has proven that traditional methods to screen and inform black women concerning breast cancer leaves much to be desired. In the early 1960's when Dr Philip Strax pioneered the first large scale screening for breast cancer (See Chapter 6), it was discovered that black women responded the least to public service announcements on the radio or television. Direct targeting by mail and telephone also produced few subscribers among black women.

Many of us who have been involved in breast cancer awareness programs know that when the black public is invited to such a gathering in a community center, black church, or other venue, the turnout is consistently sparse. Simply stated, nobody wants to go out of their way to hear about breast cancer—or any other cancer for that matter. The answer is: You must, whenever feasible, present the message to a captive audience.

For example, the Witness Project in Little Rock in which breast cancer survivors were given time during the Sunday morning church service to give their personal witness of overcoming breast cancer. At the same time those breast cancer survivors took the opportunity to urge parishioners to get a physical check up and a mammogram. They understood that their presentation during the morning service was to a *captive* audience.

Another captive audience is the African-American beauty parlor. Perhaps an even greater audience than the church. All black women do not go to church on a regular basis; but virtually all black women get to a beauty parlor from time to time. I suspect that there is something basically therapeutic and fulfilling about having the hair washed, set and styled.

Where else will black women devote half a day for an optional activity? The beauty parlor has got to be the perfect captive audience.

Someone must have thought, 'If we can just slide in a little music and a celebrity speaking on a video, perhaps we can offer a message to these women about the importance of breast cancer.' Perhaps many of you enterprisers reading this book will be inspired to set something in motion in your own community.

First you must find grant money to provide a video and television unit to present your program in participating beauty parlors. There must be funds to induce the beauty operator to play the video and pass out brochures and vouchers for low cost or no cost mammograms. Finally you must find a hospital or clinic to provide the mammograms. In this way you will be reaching a population where breast cancer has reached epidemic proportions.

Deidra Forte in Los Angeles has had some success in carrying out such a project. She and her associates understood that in every black community there is at least one beauty shop. You can get the details of how it was set up and how it was funded by calling (310) 271-7732.

In Pittsburgh, PA, a similar project is functioning. Beauty and the Breast, headed by Ms LaVerne Baker, the Minority Outreach Coordinator, Commonwealth Division of the American Cancer Society, Greater Pittsburgh Unit. They have implemented a program that reaches women at beauty parlors servicing the black community in Pittsburgh. Ms Baker is also the founder and chair of SisterReach Advisory Council. The Council is comprised of volunteers from the American Cancer Society and the Susan G Komen Foundation. Their mission is to reach more African American women concerning the importance of mammography and breast self-examination (BSE). Patrons at the participating beauty shops are given an educational packet and information about a Mammogram Voucher Program which provides payment for mammograms for uninsured and under-insured women in the Pittsburgh area.

SisterReach also sponsors other activities to reach African-American

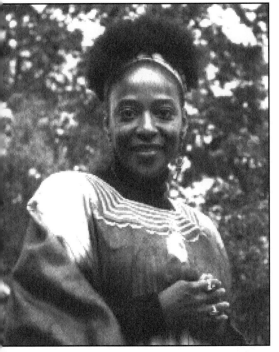

g. 10-5. La Verne Baker

women with life-saving information concerning breast cancer. Since 1995 SisterReach has held an annual breast care symposium. In April, 1998, "The Essence of Beauty: Breast Health/Black Women Health Symposium and Fashion Show" will be held, providing the latest information regarding breast cancer in the black community. This project is co-sponsored by the American Cancer society.

Since 1997 SisterReach has produced a calendar highlighting breast cancer survivors. This project is funded by the Susan G Komen. Fund.

"Race for the Cure," sponsored by SisterReach and funded by the Susan G Komen Fund on Mother's Day, 1996, is now a major event that highlights breast cancer awareness in the Pittsburgh area.

You can find out how these ideas can be exported to your community. Simply network with LaVerne Baker at (412) 261 4352 ext 112.

———

In speaking and fellowshipping with breast cancer survivors and women who've devoted time and treasure to this high calling, they have allowed me to glimpse their hopes and fears, their joy and triumph, their resolution and quiet faith. In Chapter 11 let me share some of the conversations that have inspired me. These women invite us into their homes and hearts and disclose how they confronted and overcame their own personal adversity

CHAPTER ELEVEN

HIS EYE IS ON THE SPARROW
Faith, Hope and Prayer—Breast Cancer Survivors Speak!

*t*here is a bird feeder just outside my breakfast nook that sits atop a post surrounded by dense azalea bushes. Almost every morning while lingering over my grits and coffee I get a chance to do a little bird watching; and I'm fascinated by the avian socialization and the established pecking order.

First I see the turtle doves, strutting proud and stately, chasing away each other for no apparent reason, except to establish the chain of com-

mand I suppose. Then come the blue-jays, with their loud chatter, two or three at a time, with their quick jerky moves, cocking the head, twisting the neck, jumping about, always on the alert. Next, the cardinal comes by to feed, festooned in cardinal red, always accompanied by his mate who's dressed in light brown but with a bright beak and orange headdress. The cardinal pair usually waits until the crowd has gone and then each will approach the feeder alone,

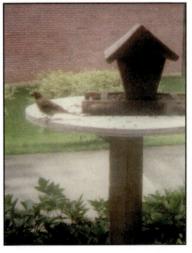

Kevin A Johnson

while their mate perches on a branch nearby. And then they switch places. I've been watching for years and this pattern remains the same.

Occasionally several black birds with their iridescent plume will flutter down squawking noisily and scattering whatever birds were there.

Sometimes canaries, decked out in yellow and black, drop by; and if I'm lucky, a woodpecker with red head, white collar and black and white speckled body will make my day.

Finally after everybody's gone, a swarm of 10 or 12 sparrows alight all of a sudden chirping and hopping about, heads a-bobbing, eyes a-darting while their vibrating beaks expertly separate the husk from the meat. The sparrow, small and scrawny, with a coat of feathers that is drab and dirty, is the scavenger, the "least of these" of birdland, cleaning up after everybody's gone. Perhaps despised by their finer feathered friends.

Are these the lowly creatures the Psalmist was thinking of when he wrote,"...His eye is on the sparrow and I know He watches me?" If God can look after the sparrow, head no bigger than a thumb nail, find shelter for him by night and lead him to food by day, surely, the Psalmist must have concluded, 'God's presence in my life will be manifest all the more.'

The hymn goes on ..."I sing because I'm happy, I sing because I'm free...For His Eye is on the Sparrow, and I know He watches me." I've met many breast cancer survivors who have a story to tell, a song to sing, if you will. They believe that the same God who takes care of the sparrow at my feeder has the power to touch their lives in a meaningful way and give them the solace and peace that we all crave and absolutely need. In these next few pages several of these women disclose in their own words, their personal response to their illness. They share with us heartfelt anxieties and fears. Their testimony of triumph and joy is based on a faith and inner strength that springs forth unrestrained by rule or reason.

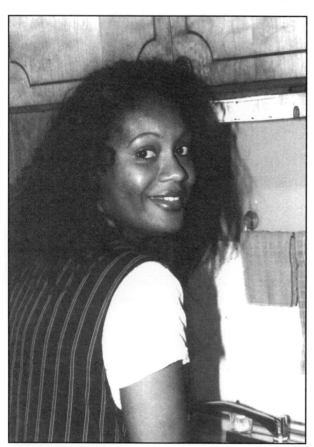

Owe'ta L Wiley

Owe'ta L Wiley, a mother of two young boys, found a thickened area in the right breast while dressing one day a few months ago. Cancer did

His Eye is on the Sparrow

not enter her mind. After all there was no family history of breast cancer. She didn't smoke or drink and she was only 33 years old.

Mrs Wiley waited a few days and then pointed out this little firm place to her husband. He suggested that she have their family doctor check it out; and in a matter of only two weeks breast cancer was diagnosed and she underwent a modified mastectomy.

Dr J: "How did you find the courage to face that diagnosis at such a young age, Mrs Wiley?"

Mrs. W: "About two months before I discovered anything, this lady was addressing a class that I was attending. She said she found joy during her bout with breast cancer. And I thought to myself, 'how could anybody find joy in cancer'. Then when I got cancer myself just two months later, I reflected back and understood what she meant. Little did I know that what that woman said about having joy would actually help me so much. I was never devastated like others might have expected, because I kept thinking about what that lady said about joy. She meant joy in knowing that God was there through it all.

"I think my strong Christian background and my husband also helped me find that joy for myself. When I first found out I had cancer, people in my family and my friends couldn't believe how well I took it; but I wanted to give God the glory in the way I adjusted to it and the way I'm handling it now. And I never ever looked at it as something bad. I look at this as something positive. It's like a song Dottie Peoples sings, "The devil meant it for bad but God meant it for good." I was apprehensive about being interviewed but then I want to help other black women and women in general, and urge them to be aware of breast cancer and get regular check-ups. I can't help other women by hiding out and just keeping it in so that's why I agreed to let it be known. The joy comes when your faith is tested and you overcome."

Dr J: "Tell me about Mr Wiley, smiling over there."

Mrs W: "My husband has been very loving. Oh yes. He has been very, very supportive. And the decision making? That was one of the hardest things I had to do. But my husband was there with me—to every doctor visit. I encourage men that have a mate faced with breast cancer to go to the office visits and ask questions, because it affects the whole family."

Dr J: "Did you get along with your doctors?"

Mrs W: "I felt real comfortable chatting with my doctor and I had no problem with hospital staff or nurses. But I did have trouble with them finding my vein (smile)."

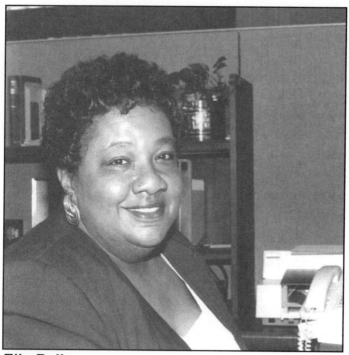

Ella Bell

Ella Bell is a dynamic professional, keen, energetic, politically astute. Well educated and a past candidate for public office.

Dr J: "How long after discovering the lump did you wait to see your doctor, Mrs Bell?"

Mrs B: "The next day. The next day. I felt this on a Sunday night. I was in the doctor's office at 8:30 on that Monday morning and had a mammogram by 11:30; and three days later I was at the surgeon's office."

Dr J: "What were the results of the mammogram? And had you had previous mammograms?"

Mrs B: "I've been getting mammograms every year and nothing ever showed up. Even my last mammogram didn't show anything, but I could still feel this knot.

"My doctor said the mammogram was negative, but the lump had to be biopsied. He found ductal carcinoma and after we discussed all of the alternatives I decided on mastectomy with immediate reconstruction with a TRAM flap (See Chapter 12). It wasn't two weeks later before I had my surgery. They said it took 14 hours, but I'm so pleased with the results. They did a wonderful job. I just wouldn't take nothing for my doctor. When he told me it was cancer, the first thing I said was, 'Is it going to kill me?'

"And he said, 'Oh no, no baby. This is early. You're in good shape. When we go in there if we find nothing in your lymph nodes, then you're in excellent shape.' You know, Dr Johnson, they took 26 lymph nodes and there was no cancer present."

Quemellar Lane is a 50 year old legislative aide employed by the Alabama Senate for the past twenty years. She drives a late model sports utility vehicle and is active in social and community affairs. While her life seems orderly and stable at present, it wasn't always that way.

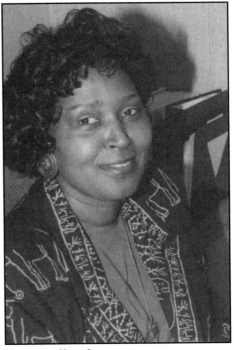

Quemellar Lane

In 1969, at age 22 Mrs Lane slightly bruised the left breast on a coffee table while playing on the floor with her toddlers. Pain and tenderness directed her hand to a lump in the breast which she ascribed to the injury. In a few days the soreness would subside but the knot in the breast remained. Indeed the lump was confirmed by her doctor some days later. The doctor ordered a mammogram, and a few days later a radical mastectomy was done with removal of the breast and the underlying muscles and extensive dissection of the armpit. She was also treated with radiation. As you can imagine those were days of deep depression for that 22-year-old mother. Dread of dying and leaving her two small children was all pervading. Her husband was far away in the Navy, on-board ship. Her mother was frightened, but provided comfort as best she could. What made her ordeal even more harrowing was that she agreed to radical surgery immediately if her biopsy was positive for cancer. She was not given any alternative. That was the state of affairs in 1969.

Mrs L: "When they took the bandages off the doctor said, 'Oh that's beautiful. I did a great job. What a beautiful scar; the surgery was a great success.' But when I looked at it I thought it was horrible. I told them not to even call my husband back from the ship. But they had to because of some regulation. He did not know how to cope with it. And I didn't either.

My greatest fear was dying. My girls were 3 and 1 ½ years old. How could I adjust to this? When my husband came home he didn't know what to say; and he began staying away from home more and more. I thought it was because I had only one breast. Naturally I went into a slump; but I finally realized I had to get over this and I had to go on and live for myself. My mom was my greatest source of strength. I had gotten away from the church after marriage so I didn't have that to help me over."

Dr J: "Were you able to stay with your husband?"

Mrs L: "Well let me tell you. Somehow, we got back together. I guess our love was strong enough to eventually overcome it. In 1975 we had another child—a son. It was a blessing. He's 21 years old now and doing well. All of my children have given me a reason to live.

"But in 1976, my cancer returned. My son was only a year old. They found spread to the bone. I was treated with radiation and they removed my ovaries. But this time my husband and I made a better adjustment. I suppose more was being said about breast cancer then, especially with prominent people being diagnosed, and women demanding more conservative treatment.

"In 1969, when I first was diagnosed, there was no Reach to Recovery Program in this area (See Chapter 12). But after my cancer was controlled in 1976 I began to volunteer to participate in the Reach to Recovery to help other black women adjust to those first days after mastectomy. Then in 1980, my aunt, my father's sister, died of breast cancer. And other women I knew had died of breast cancer. I began to feel that I was giving false hope to women when I represented the Reach to Recovery Program. It was hard for me to continue to visit black women through the American Cancer Society's Reach to Recovery Program. I was just so self-conscious because so many were dying, and I supposed some of those I talked to would also die. I began to dread going into the hospitals and talk to breast cancer patients.

"But when I did go, I tried to emphasize that patients must follow their doctor's advice; that long life is not promised to anyone, and that each day is important to be lived to the fullest.

"And that's the way I feel today. I find courage and strength from my faith in God and my husband. I feel that this was done for some rea-

His Eye is on the Sparrow

son. When I talk to people I don't want to give them false hope. I just want survivors to live as best they can day to day."

Dr J: "Have you been satisfied with your medical doctors?"

Mrs L: "I went from one doctor to another. I finally found a doctor I liked. He would examine me and do tests during my follow-up. He would take the time to listen to any little pain or complaint I had. Then he retired and I was transferred to another doctor. But I didn't like him. On my first visit, he did not examine me. I didn't say anything because I wanted to know what his mode of operation was; but I was disappointed.

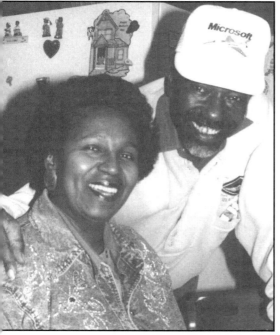

ssie Roberts and her husband

"Another doctor I had always seemed to have the black patients seen in the same examining room. Also he prescribed Depo-provera for my hot flashes in spite of my history of bone cancer. And the shot area was painful for several days, but he was very insistent that I take the shot. I simply refused. Later I read in Ebony magazine that Depo-provera was experimental for birth control, especially on black women. Needless to say, I found another physician."

Essie Roberts, has been employed as an archive technician at Maxwell Air Force Base, handling Air Force Historical Documents for the past seven years. Her husband is retired Air Force after serving 24 years. He works in the construction trade on a regular basis but was raking leaves on the balmy autumn day that I visited.

Over two years ago Mrs Roberts had a lumpectomy followed by chemotherapy for breast cancer that had spread to two lymph nodes in the axilla. She was in the habit of engaging in breast self examination (BSE) and having yearly mammograms, since she was aware that she had lumpy breasts due to fibrocystic disease. One day she came across a breast lump that was different.

Dr J: "How long did you wait to see your doctor?"

Mrs R: "Well, I had had a mammogram eleven months previously that was normal except for fibrocystic changes of course. So when I felt this lump I kept putting off seeing my doctor for about two months. But I couldn't rest. This lump just was different from the others. I knew I needed to go in. I just couldn't rest. Finally I called my doctor and she told me to come right in and have a mammogram and ultrasound. And that's what I did. My doctor called me back. I remember it was the Friday before Columbus Day. She said she wanted to refer me to a surgeon."

Dr J: "Had you told Mr Roberts of this lump and what the doctor said?"

Mrs R: "No, all this time I was just working on my own until I found out more information. I had the mammogram within two days. But it was more than two months before I could be seen by the surgeon. I was referred to the surgeon by friends at work and decided to wait to see him rather than go to the surgeon my primary doctor had recommended."

Dr J: "Did you have a needle biopsy?"

Mrs R: "No, the doctor did an open biopsy. He cut me."

Dr J: "Were you given a choice of a needle biopsy?"

Mrs R: "No, he did not give me the choice of needle biopsy. I don't remember the name of the cancer he said I had. After the biopsy he said it was a cancer; and he gave me an option of lumpectomy or mastectomy. And then he sent me to see the oncologist and radiation doctor before I had the surgery. I chose lumpectomy. Afterwards, I had chemotherapy and radiation because there was cancer in two of the lymph nodes. I had chemotherapy first. And I was sick. I lost all my hair—everywhere. I had 6 chemotherapy treatments and anywhere from six to eight weeks of radiation. I believe it was six weeks. It was five weeks of radiating the whole area and then one week of concentrated radiation over the breast. I didn't get Tamoxifen because my cancer wasn't the kind that would be helped by Tamoxifen; so no Tamoxifen was offered. Now I see the surgeon every three months for follow-up. I had a negative biopsy on the other breast a year later. I see the oncologist every four months.

"I have been pleased with the doctor. Once I felt that he was a little short and did not answer my concerns completely."

Dr J: "And you, Mr Roberts, How have you been holding up?"

Mr. R: "Well, I feel pressure from many directions and this is just another pressure. Money problems, health problems, work problems. I'm fairly pleased with my job but I'm still on temporary status, and that bothers me. I'm 52 years old now, and my wife is 50. So I'd like my work to be more stable. We've been married for 28 years."

Dr J: "I understand you've had three children."

Mr R: "The oldest teaches at Wares Ferry School. He's 27. Our oldest daughter works at Girls Inc in Memphis. She is 23."

Mrs R: "My daughter was in college and close to her finals at the University of Memphis when I had my biopsy; and I was concerned that I had to tell her this type of thing; and it was getting so close to her having her finals at the time.

"But let me tell you, Dr Johnson, I do believe strongly in God and I've leaned on it. I..I..I believe strongly in God. I believe that's what gets me through from one moment to the other one. But needless to say I don't look on this as a problem for me. You know, I know that I'm going to die one day and I don't know when; but I also realize that I've got to live, I..I..I've got to live, and I've got to live the very best that I possibly can. It hasn't held me back one way or the other so far. It's not my intention for it to hold me back."

Dr J: "Do you feel that your spirituality, your religion, your belief in God has been your main strength?"

Mr R: "Absolutely it has."

Mrs R: "I know it has."

Jessie M Williams is a dental hygienist by training, and, in fact, was the first African-American to practice in Montgomery after completing her studies at the University of Alabama Dental School in 1969. Since then she has been active in the State Dental Hygiene Program, and today she serves on the advisory committee at the Trenholm State Dental Assisting Program. She has volunteered over the years at the American Cancer Society and is an active member in her church. She has raised three children—all grown now and doing well.

Ms W: "This is a picture of my two daughters and my son. Marcia is a teacher, Shirley works for the State, and Larry is in the Navy. My children gave me this picture of them just before I went to surgery on Mother's Day last year. I had my mastectomy on Mother's Day in 1995."

Dr J: "How old were you then."

Ms W: "I was sixty-one. I had a mammogram in April and had the surgery in May. That was the first mammogram I ever had. There was no spread to my lymph nodes. Isn't that something? I got this new insurance and I was just taking advantage of it and getting myself checked out. And they found a cancer before it had spread. Now that was a blessing."

Dr J: "It was indeed. But I don't have to ask you why you waited until you were in your sixties before you had your first mammogram. It's just human nature to put things off unless you're in pain. Right?"

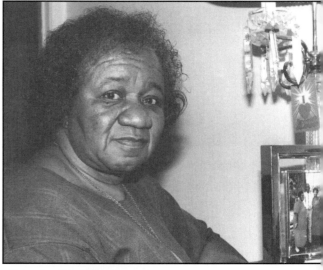

Jessie M Williams

Ms W: "I been putting my health on the back burner. But when I had good insurance I decided to take advantage and get a mammogram. My family doctor suggested it. I've been blessed to have such fine doctors.

"I retired after my breast surgery and my children take care of me, one hundred percent. My family is great to me. Of course I miss working with my dental patients. I've met so many wonderful people over the years.

"Even though I'm not working now, I stay busy. Everybody says I'm a people person, because I stay so active. In fact soon's you leave I got to go to a committee meeting.

"I took care of my mother and grandmother after they got up in years, and now my children take care of me. It's a blessing. God is able. I tell people all the time don't worry. You got to put something out there to

His Eye is on the Sparrow

get something back."

Dr J: "You've found joy, knowing that God is able. And you were blessed with good doctors too."

Ms W: "You know, the doctor who operated on me, I use to look after him when he was three years old. Now he's looking after me. I see him every three months. He checks me over and doesn't charge me a thing."

Dr J: (looking around the living room) "I see you have an organ."

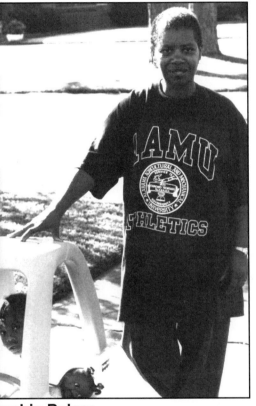

nobia Belsar

Ms W: "I had a piano that I finally gave to my granddaughter; but I came across this organ and I got such a good deal on it, I had to get it. My grand daughter and my daughter play and the kids are starting to play too. You know I have nine grand-children and three great grandchildren. There's always some music in this house. I praise the Lord for that."

Zenobia Belsar was gently pushing the FISCHER-PRICE kiddie-car down the walkway, that carried her two and a half year old grand-daughter. The sidewalks were broad and the front lawns well mani-cured by proud owners in this middle-class quiet neighborhood. Grandmother and granddaughter were having a grand time, riding, pushing and engaged in small-talk.

Dr J: "Good morning Mrs Belsar, looks like you all are having a good time. Is the baby talking much yet?"

Mrs B: "Oh yes, I don't know why she's so quiet now. Probably just shy. This child is what keeps me going ever since my surgery, Dr Johnson."

Dr J: "Tell me about your surgery."

Mrs B: "You know my surgery was two months ago. But before that I was on chemotherapy for four months before they could do my mas-tectomy because the cancer was so big. I lost all my hair. I was a GI Jane.

But it's coming back now," she smiled. "My son doesn't like me wearing a wig. He said, 'just edge it up.' "

Dr J: "I agree with your son. You're a woman of the 90's. Most of the Sisters are wearing their hair short now anyway. It's what's happening. The hair dressers can trim and style it to your satisfaction. But tell me, and I know your doctor must have asked you, why did you wait so long before seeing about yourself?"

Mrs B: "Well, I knew I had fibrocystic disease from a mammogram done in 1991, when I was 39. But I hadn't bothered to get a mammogram since then. I've never really been sick, no more than a headache. I haven't even had the flu in my whole life. And I've always been a care-giver. I took care of my mom until she died of heart failure in 1984.

"When I first noticed this lump in my right breast two years ago, in 1994, I was busy seeing about my girlfriend who had to have a hysterectomy. And then I was worried about my son who was having his own problems. So I guess I put off taking care of myself.

"I didn't feel sick. I was still getting up at 5 o'clock taking care of my children and going to work. But the knot started growing real big and there were veins and red marks on the skin and that's when I got scared.

"My sister had a breast biopsy years ago but it wasn't cancer. I don't have any family history of cancer. So I was hoping for the best until the biopsy came back. After the biopsy showed cancer, my doctor looked at me and he said, 'I can look at you and I know you're in shock'. He said, 'Darling it hurts me more to tell you this than for you to receive it. You should have come to me', and I said, 'I probably should have. But I was feeling so good.' "

"My girlfriend brought me a bible and underlined it. I get strength from reading my bible. I believe Dr Johnson that through his stripes I will be saved. I'm a good person and I know that He will not put anything more on me than I can bear. I've had a lot to contend with. My son, this grand baby, my momma dying, and so many personal problems. They just keep coming and coming.

"Some people would throw up their hands. But my grand baby keeps me going. And my faith in God keeps me going. My grand baby pats my chest and says, 'This side sore mamma?' If I say, 'Yes', she'll pat the

His Eye is on the Sparrow

other side and say, 'This side not sore.' She really keeps me going.

"The biggest thing I have now is just surges of heat and night sweats. I sweat so bad I have to get up at night and change. Isn't there something I can get for that?"

Ezetta Howard is a thirty-seven year old breast cancer survivor of two years. She counts it fortunate to be employed at a local school for retarded citizens as a bus driver.

When Ezetta was 33 years old she went to a clinic during "Breast Cancer Awareness Month" for a mammogram, because her mother and sister had had breast cancer. But even with that family history she was turned away and told to wait until she was 35 before seeking a mammogram. Within the next 18 months Ms Howard found a breast lump. The doctor said it was a cyst and drained it. But it came right back in two weeks. So the doctor did a biopsy, and it showed breast cancer. Then he did a mastectomy at the same time, and later chemotherapy was prescribed.

Ms H: "I didn't lose my hair though. The nurse told me to not use any chemicals in my hair. Let it go natural. So I let it go nappy natural. Just kept it oiled, and that's what saved it."

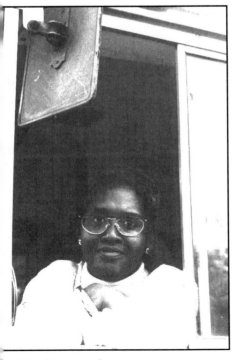

Ezetta Howard

Dr J: "How did you get through all this, and how are you doing now?"

Mrs H: "Well, my children helped me a lot. My son's 19 now. And I have two teenage daughters. They helped. Changing my bandages and helping around the house. I lost my job at Captain D's after my surgery. They wouldn't hire me back, and I got real depressed. For a while I had to go to Mental Health. I didn't go out much at all. My social life was down. But when I found this job working with the retarded, it worked out fine. I believe it was a blessing in disguise. I feel like I'm working with someone who needs me. By me having cancer and all, I can kind of relate to these retarded people who need someone."

Nina Beauchamp with a doctorate in Human Development has been teaching at a State technical college for the past fifteen years. Twenty years ago at the age of 40 during one of her periodic self-breast examinations she discovered a lump.

Dr B: "My husband was helping me examine myself and we noticed this little knot. I made an appointment and saw my doctor two days later. He suggested a biopsy and said if the biopsy were malignant they would go on and do a modified mastectomy. And that's what happened. At first I was completely depressed. But my husband and my mother helped me get through it. I had two little boys, so I was pretty worried.

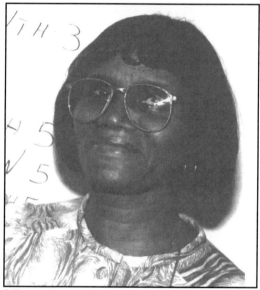

Nina Beauchamp

Dr J: "Did you have any radiation or chemotherapy."

Dr B: "No I didn't at that time. Then in 1979, three years later, I began having this horrible backache. My doctor couldn't find anything. I had all kinds of tests. Finally I went to another doctor and they did a spinal tap, a myelogram, and there it was. The cancer had metastasized to my spine. And then they recommended chemo and radiation. They thought that it had gone too far to hope for a cure, but they wanted to make me comfortable. This was a tough time. I was so sick from chemo. I lost all my hair. It was so devastating to look in the mirror——and there I'd be with no hair.

"But my husband, daily, everyday, told me I was pretty. We had two small sons and my husband would tell them, 'Mommie is so beautiful.' All the time he would tell me, 'I'm so glad I married you.' Can you imagine that?

"The doctor said there was nothing more to do. My mother said, 'Don't worry about it. I've prayed and the Lord says you're going to live'. And she just continued to say that. She had the faith. She said, 'No. You

His Eye is on the Sparrow

are not going to die'. And she said that over and over again. I just thought she was in a state of denial. Now don't get me wrong. I believe in the Lord but I told my mother that if I live it's okay and if I don't live it's still okay because I'll be just going on to glory so it doesn't matter. It's really okay.

"I tried to keep it a secret. But it was too much of a burden for my husband. He said that if something happened to me, my family, my brothers and sisters, would never forgive him. So he called them, all over the country, to let them know how sick I was. At Christmas time they all came. By that time I was bedridden just about. I was vomiting all the time. I couldn't eat. I had got down to a hundred pounds. It was horrible. I kept the religious stations on all the time. One time Earnest Ainsley, the evangelist, was on the television and it was announced that he was coming to Birmingham. My husband cried and said that he was going to take me to see him. But I was so sick. He made a bed in the back seat and we drove to my mother's house in Clanton. Then my husband, my sister and my mother took me on to Birmingham.

"This big auditorium. You know how he's praying for folks. Finally he said, 'Everybody who has cancer, I want you to come up'. My husband carried me up to the front. The evangelist was just going down the line praying for each one and touching them on the head. He touched me on the head and I just went out. They call it, 'slain in the spirit'. You know, when I would see people falling out on stage on TV I use to say, 'you know they ought to quit'."

Dr J: "Like on Benny Hinn?"

Dr B: "That's right. But I really went out. My sister thought he kind of pushed me over, me being so weak. But I really went out. Then he touched my husband and he went out too. It was really something. I can't explain it.

"Well, we drove back to Montgomery and the next day I started getting stronger. I had not been out of the house for weeks. But I went out in the yard the day after we got back home. My neighbor looked out the window and thought I was a ghost, I looked so bad. But everyday I got stronger and stronger. I went back to my doctor and asked to have another myelogram and he said to wait three months. Because, I guess, he thought I'd be disappointed. So I waited. And then I had another myelogram. My doctor called me and said, 'Nina, the cancer is gone. The cancer is gone.' You can imagine how excited my husband and I were. My doctor told me it was a miracle. He had absolutely no idea how it worked.

"My son is now 30. When he was a growing up, he decided he wanted to be an oncologist, a cancer doctor. We always figured it was because he was so worried about me when he was little and I had cancer, that he wanted to be a doctor to help me. So now, do you know, he's actually finished medical school. Isn't it amazing how God works. And I'm blessed with another son too. My younger son is a Navy man with a wonderful family. They are *both* wonderful sons."

Dr J: "Your experience is just a testament that God is real. And He is able."

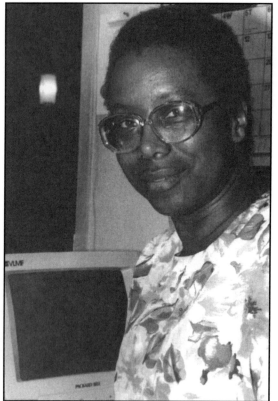

Johnnie Sellers

Dr B: "He sure is able. I've been married for 35 years. Thank God we are very compatible. God has given me time over these past 20 years; and everyday I try to use it wisely."

Remember that song.."You've go to Accent—tuate the positive! Elim—minate the negative! Latch on to the affirmative! And don't mess with Mister in between?" Well, that's **Johnnie Sellers**. Her smile is quick and easy and when she speaks her eyes simply sparkle. Her voice fills the room with sunshine and laughter. Upbeat, optimistic. Completely at home with herself.

Johnnie Sellers is a special person. One of God's children living the life, not just talking the talk. She didn't have a lot to say about her religion but there was no mistake in my mind, this lady knew where she was, and where her God was. She knew she was safe and secure from all alarm.

The evening I visited her working at the church office, she was busy typing names into the computer.

Dr J: "How long will you be here tonight, Mrs Sellers?"

Mrs S: " 'til I'm through," she laughed. "I've got to make a list of the deacon board, the trustee board and the board of christian education. And these lists must be ready for the conference Saturday. But my regular job is to take the Sunday collection envelopes and record each name and amount given into the computer so that there is a record of giving for each member. I suppose I'll be here about three more hours."

I thought to myself, 'This lady is really too busy to waste time with me'. But she was able to chat and laugh and still keep on working. I enjoyed our visit. I was mindful that she was doing a job for the church she loved, but still wanted to tell some of the story that brought me to her office this night.

Dr J: "How old were you when you were diagnosed with breast cancer?"

Mrs S: "Let's see, it goes back a ways. I'm 48 now. Let's see, it goes back to when I was 33. I found this knot in my breast. I knew right away it was probably a cancer. I noticed the lump and I also had a cloudy discharge from my breast. I knew it was probably a cancer, but my doctor thought it most likely wasn't because I was so young I suppose. But I had several aunts with breast cancer. It's not something I was afraid of. It's something I anticipated.

"I had the biopsy and mastectomy at the same time. No chemotherapy. Then two years later I found cancer in my remaining breast, so I had that side done. Mastectomy. That was 12 years ago. I didn't want any lumpectomy and radiation. I worried about them missing something if any breast was left behind. When I was a little girl I had a cousin who had a mastectomy and radiation and I could see the burn marks in the skin. So I didn't want any parts of radiation.

"When I turned 48 the cancer came back. I just finished chemotherapy a few weeks ago, and Dr Johnson, was I sick. My Lord! I lost all my hair. And I got so small. When I came back to church, people were telling me how small I was. At first that chemo took my appetite. But after a while I guess I got used to the chemo and my appetite came back. I have a friend who's a member of this church, and she would cook and bring me food everyday; and I started eating and eating and I kept eating. I had bought some clothes for this little frame I thought I was going to keep. After a month I couldn't fit in them clothes. So I really picked up my weight. And I'm feeling fine now. I've been back teaching for the past three months. You see my hair is growing back but I'm keeping it trimmed. I really like it short. How do you like it now?"

Dr J: "I think it looks great. Let me take one more picture."

She laughed and made a comic pose and then for a brief moment she was serious, peering into my face over her glasses.

Mrs S: "You know, it's just a blessing to be up and about."
Like other survivors she, too, had found joy.

Carrie Nelson-Hale was 36 years old when she found a lump in the right breast while taking a shower.

Mrs H: "My breasts are small and I could see this little protrusion sticking out when I raised my arm overhead. I got out of the shower, dried down, and woke my husband immediately. He's a doctor and he examined me. He didn't think it was anything, but we agreed that I should have it examined further.

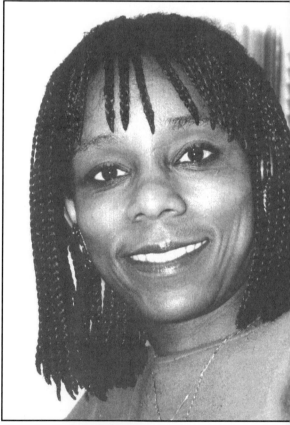

Carrie Nelson-Hale

"I was working as a social worker at this hospital so I went to one of the attending surgeons. I told him I had had a mammogram the year before and it was alright. He said I needed a biopsy. I went to four different doctors. Three advised me to have a biopsy and immediate mastectomy if the biopsy was positive. One doctor advised observing the lump for six months."

Dr J: "Did they advise repeat mammogram?"

Mrs H: "No. This happened in 1990. I asked about lumpectomy and no doctor was willing to consider that as an alternative. Even my husband thought mastectomy was best and that kind of swayed me."

Dr J: "You say you were in social work?"

Mrs H: "I got my undergraduate degree from Michigan State and then went to the University of South Carolina for my Masters. Then I went back to Michigan to work. That's where I met my husband.

"Anyway, when I awoke from surgery the breast was removed. They said there was no spread and I didn't get radiation or chemotherapy. But I wondered about that.

Dr J: "I suspect those were some tough days."

Mrs H: "They were."

Dr J: "How did you manage those days? What helped you to get through those times? Did you somehow reach down inside?"

Mrs H: "Well——my faith. I've always had a strong faith in God."

Dr J: "So you kind of came up in the church?"

Mrs H: "Not 'kind of'," she laughed. "My grandmother was Pentecostal and my parents were southern Baptists, so I had a thorough indoctrination. I grew up in a town called Ninety-six, South Carolina. Small and close knit. So when I got up a little I went away to school.

"After I had cancer my religion became part of my 'treatment team'. I also used imagery along with prayer. I would visualize the good cells killing the cancer cells.

"And then I keep busy working in the community making people aware of the importance of breast cancer detection. You know I've organized breast cancer survivors to spread information and encourage regular mammograms.

I met **Debbie Norrell** in Pittsburgh two years ago when she served as the Mistress of Ceremonies at a fashion show. Interestingly, all the participants in that fashion show were breast cancer survivors, ranging in age from the late twenties to sixty-something. The show was a smashing success, but in the mind of many it was the chic moderator, Debbie Norrell,

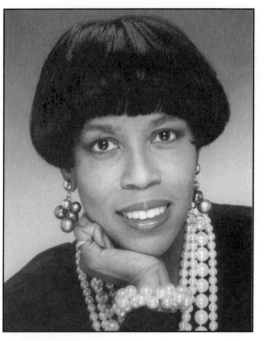
Debbie Norrell

who put the zing into the affair that made it a memorable event.

Later I learned that Debbie, herself, was a five year breast cancer survivor. At age 37, one day, she simply felt tired and below par. Nothing to do with the breast. Just more tired than usual after an afternoon of shopping. However, when she went in for a general exam, her doctor pointed out a discreet nodule just below her collar bone in the upper part of her breast. A core needle biopsy confirmed the suspicion of breast cancer; and this was followed by lumpectomy, radiation and long-term Tamoxifen.

This ordeal has not slowed Debbie, who looks inward for support and strength. Family and loved ones are fine but ultimately "you have to keep on going for yourself". Two weeks after surgery she was auditioning for a movie. She has been doing voice overs and commercials and is an aspiring actress. Debbie also has a daily talk show on radio station WAMO in Pittsburgh.

Her joy comes from using her talent and talk show to keep the community informed about political, societal, and health issues.

Incidently, you can look for Debbie Norrell in the movie, "Desperate Measures".

All of these women have remained steadfast, focused on their faith and innate strength. They keep busy taking care of their families, pursuing worthwhile goals, and taking on the task of informing others on the importance of breast self-examination and mammography.

They remain attuned to carrying out everyday chores and yet relishing the silver threads of joy that intertwine and highlight their lives. Their joy has been burnished by adversity, pain, and victory. It's a joy that gives meaning and purpose to each day. These survivors continue to persevere as each one witnesses the pageantry of life unfolding in their individual circumstance.

Even when the outlook was equivocal at best, these women were willing to accept and adjust, and remain steadfast. Somehow, without forming the words or defining the terms these survivors combined the practical, the philosophical, and the spiritual to find a peace of mind and inner 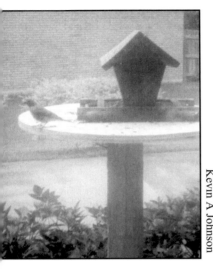 power to move on. As some women related their experiences to me, their voices rising in testimony, I relived my own early days, listening to Charlie Mae Haynes singing in the Third Baptist Church where I came of age in San Francisco—"I sing because I'm happy, I sing because I'm free, For His eye is on the sparrow and I know He watches me."

Breast cancer survivors, through their testimonials, ignite within their listeners a spark, that enables the listeners to clearly see and successfully confront their own personal challenges.

Kevin A Johnson

———

In the next chapter I shall speak to the notion—that the mission of life can indeed be fulfilled—-with the help of agencies devoted to rehabilitation, with choices of chemotherapy and plastic surgery, and with the comforting support of loved ones. And most of all because of the discovery of an inexplicable joy within, that can be harnessed, and amplified, and directed.

Therefore we are always confident, knowing that, while we are at home in the body, we are absent from the Lord.

(For we walk by faith, not by sight);

We are confident, I say, and rather to be absent from the body, and to be present with the Lord.

II Corinthians 6:8

CHAPTER TWELVE

LIGHTS, CAMERA, ACTION!
The Show Must Go On

S ome years ago I made a house call on Abby Lincoln, who was in town for a singing engagement. In those days doctors made house calls, so it was only a few minutes before I was knocking on her hotel door, black bag in hand. I was greeted by an obviously ill lady, caught up in cough and sputter. The cool San Francisco fog had given her a bad cold. Unable to talk, she just waved me in.

"You're Doctor Johnson, right?," she asked with a gravelly voice, heading back to bed. "Thanks for coming." Her voice was hoarse. Her eyes were red. She coughed into Kleenex and blew her nose. The lady was sick.

"I've been coughing all day."

I opened my bag and took out my stethoscope and penlight; and wrapped a blood pressure cuff in place. Blood pressure was fine. Heart normal. But the throat was red, and the lungs congested. Her temperature was slightly elevated.

Abby's eyes looked at me questioning. "Just a bad cold, right?"

"Looks like bronchitis on the way to pneumonia, and maybe a strep throat," I responded. "You need bed rest and medication. In a few days I think you'll be okay. For now you'll have to stay put. I don't think you're used to this San Francisco weather."

She looked at me gloomily. "Doctor it's just seven o'clock. My first show is at ten. Can't you give me something? The show's got to go on," she pleaded.

I gave her an injection of antibiotic and called in three prescriptions to be delivered. I admired her drive; but doing a show was out of the question.

Breast Cancer / Black Woman

177

"What do you say Doctor Johnson? I've got to sing tonight. I've just got to."

"Sure I understand. But if you're not up to it, just get your medicine, stay in bed, and rest."

A few pleasantries and I was gone. In my mind I knew there was no way Abby would perform that night. No way.

I have been told, and do in part believe, that through rain and snow, through flood and fire, the mail must go through. The mail is essential. But did the show have to go on? Even in spite of illness? Was the show in the same category as the mail?

Later that night I happened to drop by the club where Abby was supposed to sing. Even though I knew Abby wouldn't be there, the jazz combo had been playing to rave revues. And I thought I'd take a little R and R, and check them out. As I made my way into the nightclub the lights were dimming as the spotlight sent a shaft of bright through the haze. A rotund balding gentleman on stage in formal attire was making an announcement. I caught the gist through the crowd noise. "Ladies and gentlemen...what you've been waiting for....Miss Abby Lincoln!"

Say what! I couldn't believe it. But seeing was believing. The spotlight illuminated the edge of the platform and indeed—it was Abby Lincoln. The light caught her smile—-sparkling and provocative. Her movements were crisp and animated; her eyes danced and twinkled as the spot light captured the toss of her head and the rhythm in her step. She wore a frilly red blouse and black cigarette pants with spike heels. Transformed. Stepping high to the music. And she proceeded to dance *and* sing. Her voice was a bit coarse and she cleared her throat a couple of times. But the radiant smile never wavered. There were no excuses about not feeling up to par. The crowd loved her and she loved the crowd. The jazz band was energized by her dance and song. Abby worked the house and just did her thing for the next 30 minutes. Everybody clapped, stomped, and bellowed; and I just sat back in disbelief. It was unreal.

What is this business about the 'show must go on?' Is there something to it after all? I knew Abby had to be feeling terrible. How did she pull it off? It had to be sheer will power—mind over matter. Dedicated to the performance. Unwilling to let her audience or herself down. I could hear a little rasp in her voice and perhaps her eyes were a bit red. But who cared. The lady went on and simply took care of business.

Now that I think about it, I've seen something like that in my own family and you've seen it too. Struggling against one adversity after another for a greater purpose. In fact we see it around us all the time. Folks working long hours in spite of pain. Old women standing on arthritic knees cooking and cleaning house for little or nothing—maybe bringing home a covered dish of leftovers—but still trying to keep it together. They are all part of the notion that the 'show must go on'.

Even after serious illness such as breast cancer or whatever foul circumstance that should befall, life must still go on. Doctors and nurses, with all of their skill, are important; but they play only minor roles. If there is support from family and friends, so much the better. But when all is said and done, it is you the patient, the woman, who must rise up, take center stage and face the turmoil of tomorrow. This is your life.

You may ask, "How is this possible? This is not the flu or arthritis! I've just lost my breast and I still may not be cured!"

Well it is possible. I've seen others overcome, and so can you. Here's how to get started. It's the same formula you use when facing any calamity or severe test. First of all, focus carefully on whatever blessings and good fortune you *do* have. Without even thinking very hard you will begin to realize first one blessing after another. There always seems to be someone a little worse off who is surviving and overcoming some handicap. You'll discover you can be truly thankful for whatever you have, great or small. Then, start praying on a regular basis for courage and strength and faith, and then act!

Go into action by directing your mind on what to think. My father used to tell me, 'Think big and you'll be big. Think small and you'll be small'. You still have free will, so think good thoughts, do good deeds, control your actions, even your tone of voice as you relate to your family and friends. Concentrate on being polite towards family, friends, casual acquaintances, strangers and even bill collectors. The power of the tongue has the capacity to bring a sense of inner peace. The more sunshine you share with others, the more light and warmth will be reflected towards you. And this will nurture your life and your survival.

The entertainer, Lola Falana, said it best. When faced with a life threatening illness, she remarked, "I'm not cured, but I'm healed." In other words she was saying, "I've come to terms with my life. God is always good and He will be with me no matter what happens."

If you want to be happy, act happy. If you want to be strong, then act strong. Always search for the best part of any circumstance. You will find that if you act enthusiastic, you will actually become enthusiastic; and those supporting players around you will reflect your attitude and add to your strength and fortitude.

No, you are not superwoman by any means and there are sure to be moments of despair. However, you have a mind with the ability to direct and channel your thoughts! You can compel the mind to think positively, or allow it to drift negatively. Just try it. The mind is the most important part of the body. All other parts serve to keep it functioning. If you were paralyzed from the neck down, you could still be creative. Certainly you can be creative and fulfilled without an arm or a leg, or a breast. Even without the ability to see, one can be productive and creative. Set your thoughts into action, positive action! Never forget that you are the star of the show, and the show must go on, no matter if you've been completely cured or the cord of life has simply been lengthened for a season.

Adjustment following breast cancer treatment means not only physical recovery, but emotional healing as well. Too often, it means learning to live with incurable disease. You must minimize the brooding and self-pity. Read books of inspiration. Read of people who've overcome obstacles. Read Psalms and Job, Ecclesiastes and Proverbs. Read about Jesus and Paul. Without a doubt you will find power hidden deep inside that you didn't know existed. Read the Bible with the purpose of inspiration. This is a time in life for reflection and re-evaluation, a time to set new goals. A time for the mind to go into action.

Once you thank God for what you do have, you automatically turn a switch in the mind from negative despair to positive hope. It works. And once you're on the road to a positive frame of mind, you're ready for rehabilitation and moving on to new pursuits. This is where the medical professionals play a role.

Lights, Camera, Action!

REACH TO RECOVERY

The Reach to Recovery Program of the American Cancer Society has given incalculable assistance in the emotional readjustment of the post-mastectomy patient. This is a program of volunteers who visit mastectomy patients several days after surgery with helpful comments and answers to those 'woman to woman' questions.

All volunteers have had the same operation and are matched as nearly as possible with the patient's ethnic background, age, education and economic status. Black breast cancer survivors in many sections of the country are cooperating with the American Cancer Society and providing volunteers to counsel with recently treated black patients.

In 1976 the Reach to Recovery launched their Man-to-Man program in which a husband of a post-mastectomy patient was available to speak by phone on issues that were not strictly medical. This program was designed to allow husbands whose wives were recently operated, to talk with men who had been through the same experience.

In 1996, the **Breast Cancer Resource Committee** in Washington, DC, (See Chapter 10) launched a program dedicated to involving black men in getting the message out to the black women in their lives. This reflects the importance of involving the whole family in the fight against breast cancer. It can only enhance the Reach to Recovery Program.

The idea of one woman with a mastectomy reaching out to lend emotional support to another who had just undergone similar surgery was put forth by Mrs. Teresa Lasser in 1952 following her own mastectomy. She saw the special need for one woman to reach out to another in such a time of stress. In 1969 the American Cancer Society adopted Mrs. Lasser's program and called it "Reach to Recovery". Over the years millions of women have been helped.

Volunteers bring helpful pamphlets and brochures. They demonstrate exercises and often provide a temporary prosthesis to be worn home from the hospital.

Post-mastectomy volunteers give encouragement as no other group can, for they are living proof of what the patient can attain. The Reach to Recovery volunteer can relate her own moment of depression and personal difficulties. Personal vignettes and suggestions for overcoming barriers can be discussed. The volunteer can encourage the patient to exercise and warn against shoulder stiffness. Obviously these volunteers must be carefully selected and trained. They are well groomed, bright and outgoing. Ordinarily no more than three hospital visits are made, and only with the approval of the attending physician. In their own unique way they tell the patient, "You are the show, and the show must go on."

In the black community innovative programs associated with the American Cancer Society, the Susan G Komen Fund have been forged by locally inspired black women. Chapter Ten provides some examples of these programs.

REHABILITATION AND COMPLICATIONS

Even before treatment is scheduled, the physician is expected to discuss and explain in some detail the type of treatment (surgery, radiation and/or chemotherapy) he believes is preferable in any particular case. If you or a loved one are being counseled, be sure you do not feel rushed and that all questions are answered to your satisfaction. If surgery is the option, inquire about radiation. If radiation is suggested be certain that all the surgical options are fully discussed. A family member, perhaps a daughter or husband, or a trusted friend should be with you to help with the questions since it is often difficult to remember everything you wish to ask. So while you're thinking, your husband or son can join the discussion. If a biopsy has been done, this is the time to discuss the results and implications for prognosis. In these preliminary talks you also want to know the anticipated problems and complications to be faced while recuperating.

For example, one may expect some tightness over the chest wall if a mastectomy has been performed. Deep breathing exercises to inflate the compressed lung are important. Occasionally a chronic cough develops. This is a good time for smokers to stop smoking.

There may also be arm swelling and shoulder stiffness in many patients. Early swelling may be due to interruption of the lymph channels that serve the arm, or infection at the operative site. Significant swelling is usually temporary and with early physical therapy it generally subsides. In one study about 25 percent of women who had extensive axillary dissection, arm swelling was serious and required vigorous sustained treatment including an elastic arm sleeve and antibiotics. In another study, Dr Judith Headley of the M.D. Anderson Hospital, Houston, found that of 89 patients who developed serious swelling, only 55 percent had received physical therapy. In 189 patients who did receive post-operative physical therapy only 33 percent had significant arm swelling.[1]

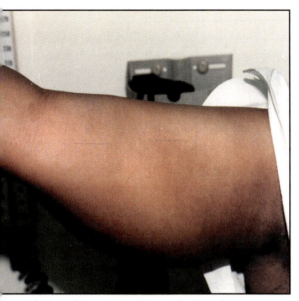

g. 12-1. **Arm swelling following mastctomy. This condition is frequently een after mastectomy, but it usually bsides with time. Occasionally it persts to some extent and rarely it can be capacitating.**

In a small fraction of patients the swelling becomes incapacitating. If neglected the arm can swell three to five times that of the normal arm and become a useless appendage. Very rarely, cancer of the lymph channels in the arm (lymphangiosarcoma) will result with dire consequences.

The patient's arm must be carefully protected after breast surgery. The shoulder must be exercised during the immediate post-operative period and the arm elevated on a pillow when sleeping. One should not allow the arm to be used for taking blood samples or checking blood pressure, even after full recovery. Any minor injury to the fingers or hand should be attended to immediately. Sometimes oral medication to remove fluid and weight loss through diet control are helpful measures to control arm swelling.

Shoulder stiffness is due to inactivity because of pain and fear. If exercise is delayed, early scar tissue sets in after a few days, further restricting arm motion and ultimately leading to contractions. Often the doctor will arrange for the patient to visit a physical therapy clinic, where a therapist can outline a useful program. It is gratifying to follow the patient's response once she understands what is required.

With the almost complete elimination of radical mastectomies in favor of the modified surgery, which leaves the large chest muscles intact, the shoulder stiffness is less of a problem. I also expect that fewer cases of severe arm edema (swelling) will be seen in the future since the modified surgery requires less dissection of the axilla.

Other complications to be aware of are caused by radiation. Depending on where the beam is directed one can sustain injury to nerves in the axilla (armpit) leading to loss of function of the arm or hand. If radiation is directed to the chest wall there can be damage to the heart, lung, or ribs. Some patients have a persistent sore throat following radiation treatment that can last for weeks or months. Every effort is taken to prevent radiation complications. With newer techniques and better equipment these problems have been minimized. Severe nerve injury is largely a thing of the past, but radiation injury to the lung is still all too frequent.

PALLIATIVE TREATMENT OPTIONS

Palliative treatment is used in those cancer patients that can not be cured. The purpose of palliation is to relieve pain, bring comfort and extend life. For example, in years past, surgical removal of the ovaries followed by surgical removal of the adrenal glands or the hypophysis was carried out with frequent lengthening of life. Today, Tamoxifen, in most cases, has usurped those radical interventions. Chemotherapy and radiation are still used to control pain and extend life. These treatment methods must be weighed in the balance of benefit versus complications.

Surgery to remove the ovaries in my opinion is less hazardous than radiation because of possible radiation damage to the intestines and other organs which can pose far reaching complications.

Chemotherapy, used for both palliation and along with surgery to effect cure, can have significant complications such as loss of appetite, nausea and vomiting, and hair loss. The nausea usually subsides over time; and hair loss can often be prevented or delayed by the use of ice compresses and scalp tourniquet. By using a combination of chemotherapeutic drugs the dosage can be kept low and side effects avoided or minimized. The most serious complication of chemotherapy is bone marrow depression which can be irreversible.

The anti-estrogen, Tamoxifen, is finding a good deal of usefulness following the work of Dr Bernard Fisher and his colleagues.[2] It is being used widely in older women and in younger women with certain criteria. Often standard chemotherapy is also employed at the same time. See Chapter 9 for a discussion of anti-estrogen medication, chemotherapy and hormonal therapy.

PLASTIC SURGERY

Breast reconstruction following mastectomy means devising some method of reconstructing a mound to replace the breast tissue that has been removed.

The TRAM (transverse rectus abdominis myocutaneous) flap:

This plastic surgery intervention is accomplished by a pedicle of tissue being brought forward from the back, or it may mean a graft taken from the lower abdomen. It is most often recommended for women who have a deficient amount of skin and soft tissue on the anterior chest and more than an ample supply of such tissue in the

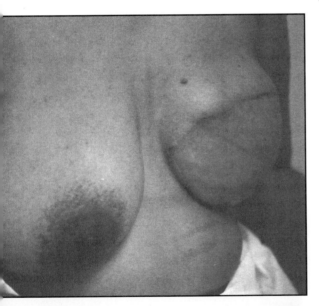
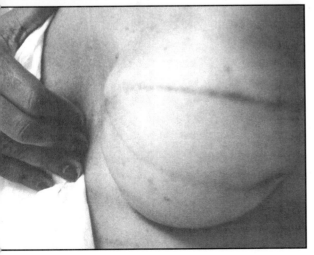

Figs. 12-2 / 12-3. The TRAM FLAP. Muscle and fat tissue can be shifted to the chest from the abdomen or flank and form an excellent breast mound that allows proper fitting of clothes as well as enhancing self-esteem in many patients.

lower abdomen. The tissue is simply swung upward to the chest wall. The obvious advantages are the avoidance of prosthetic material (silicone), and the 'tummy tuck' that is part of the procedure. A nipple complex can be fashioned some two to three months later if desired.

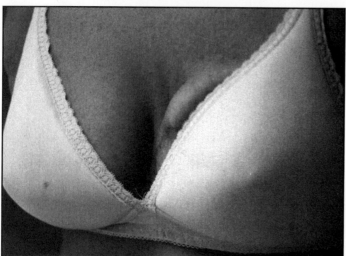

Fig. 12-4. TRAM FLAP fits well into the bra. Plastic Surgery was performed at time of mastectomy. There has been no complications and the patient is well pleased.

Although some surgeons pursue a course of immediate plastic repair at the time of initial breast amputation to lessen the psychological damage and avoid a later surgery. I would advise, if the plastic surgery is not done immediately, to wait at least six to eight months before a plastic procedure is attempted. This allows softening of scar tissue and full recovery from the cancer operation.

If plastic reconstruction is primarily undertaken to ease a sense of loss, there is a risk that the results can be less than optimal; and some women are even more distressed and fearful of facing family and spouse if the expectations of plastic surgery fall short. Therefore, it is important that a woman pause and comprehend in detail all of the possible hazards and what the operation will and will not accomplish. The patient must understand in no uncertain terms that the purpose of plastic surgery is merely to provide a breast mound suitable to hold a comfortably fitted brassiere, to allow the proper fitting of clothes and to provide some semblance of balance and symmetry.

Insist that the plastic surgical procedure and results be illustrated with drawings, photographs, and if possible by former patients. It would be helpful to talk to former patients who were happy with the outcome of plastic surgery as well as those women who were disappointed. If possible all sides of the issue should be examined. The prudent surgeon will avoid the *hard sell* or claim that plastic surgery can accomplish what it cannot. Remember, detectable wide spread metastasis or more than four axillary nodes positive for cancer argue against elective plastic surgery.

With all of these precautionary considerations, many women go ahead with plastic reconstruction immediately after mastectomy and are extremely pleased with the results.

Tissue Expander Technique

Not only may the plastic surgeon elect to use muscle and skin flaps from the back, abdomen, or buttocks, but a tissue expander technique may be used. In that method a fluid-filled plastic container is slipped under the operative site and over a matter of weeks slowly expanded by increasing the fluid in the container by pumping in saline (salt solution) to expand the tissue.

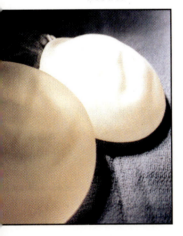

Silicone Implants

Before 1970, silicone, a synthetic oily clear liquid had been used to enlarge the female breast by direct injection. It found a market among entertainers and enjoyed a brief period of popularity. However, the free silicone in the tissue caused inflammation and pain in some cases. Abscess formation and draining ulcers were reported.

Then in the early 1970's silicone was sealed in plastic containers and placed under the breast tissue for breast augmentation. It was initially found to be quite acceptable

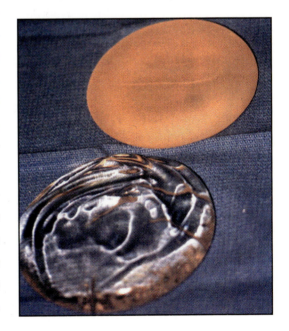

Fig. 12-5A/5B. Silicone contained in plastic containers that are either smooth or textured. Textured containers are used to prevent sliding out of place after placement.

with little side effect. From there it seemed plausible to suggest the use of contained silicone to reconstruct the breast after mastectomy. However, the operative principles had to be worked out. The guidelines for its application had to be written. Often the defect was enormous after radical mastectomy with the removal of such a large segment of tissue and muscle. So much skin was removed, that only a thin layer of tissue scarred to the ribs was left for the plastic surgeon. The

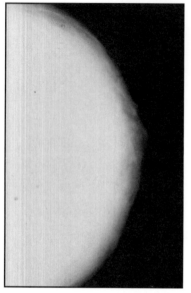

medical profession had accepted the scar and tragic cosmetic results for generations in the attempt to cure with radical cancer surgery. Obviously the non-pliable skin and tissue following such surgery was not inclined to stretch over a plastic implant.

By 1975 Americans were complaining of the mutilation of radical mastectomy and modified mastectomy was becoming more and more favored with more tissue left for plastic reconstruction and silicone implantation.

By 1990 techniques were so improved that a growing number of patients were requesting reconstruction following immediately after modified radical mastectomy. Insurance carriers provided coverage making breast reconstruction available for a wider range of women.

Fig. 12-6. Mammogram showing Silicone implant. Note the thin rim of breast tissue in front of the silicone. Detecting breast cancer in a breast that is so distorted makes it difficult to detect breast cancer. Even with special techniques, a third of the breast is not visible. BSE is not reliable.

Assemblywoman Maxine Waters (who has since become a Congresswoman) in California had written enabling legislation in 1980 that directed insurance carriers to cover reconstructive breast surgery following breast cancer surgery (AB 3548); and in 1984 Assemblywoman Waters introduced a bill directed at Medicaid (AB 2440) to provide the means to make this surgery also available to indigent patients.

Then in 1992, a moratorium was levied against further use of silicone implants while investigations were begun to sort out the risks and complications. In 1997 the moratorium against silicone was still in effect. Women were complaining that silicone was directly related to the occurrence of connective tissue disease. The issue remains undecided.

However, we *do* know that silicone breast implantation may lead to contracture and scarring. Of the 2 million women who have had silicone

Lights, Camera, Action!

implants, capsular contracture rate as high as 74 percent has been reported, with obvious deformity and dissatisfaction.**3** In another series, capsular contracture was found in 50 percent of cases. Dislocation of the silicone implant as well as leakage of the gel are also potentially serious problems that may cause irritation and inflammation.**4**

It should be understood, however, that saline implants also have complications. Not only are there problems of the implant contracting and

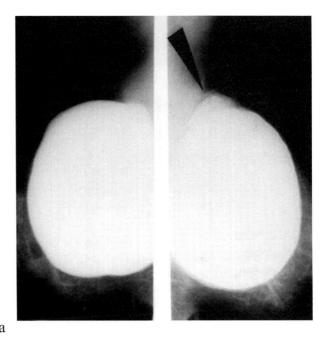

Fig12-7. Breast X-ray with silicone leak. This is a common problem that may occur several years after surgery.

moving towards the axilla, there is also a deflation rate of 16 percent due to slow leakage.**5**

If you are considering silicone or a saline implant, remember that, because under the best of circumstances there are definite precautions to observe, and complications to anticipate, the pros and cons should be discussed *before* mastectomy.

Immediate post-operative problems include bleeding into the operative site requiring drainage and perhaps re-operation. One must understand that infection, abscess and skin sloughing are all possible—even distortion and extrusion of the implant. There is still some controversy on how to handle the scar tissue forming around the implant which sometimes requires more surgery. Anchoring the prosthesis to the chest wall can also be a problem. When done properly there is still a tendency for the implant to slide towards the axilla.

In 1996 it was reported that one year after mastectomy followed by reconstructive surgery 49 percent of the women reported chronic pain in the breast. If silicone implants were used for breast enlargement (augmentation) chronic pain was noted in 53 percent of women one year after surgery.[6]

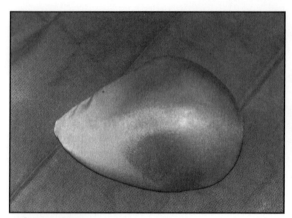
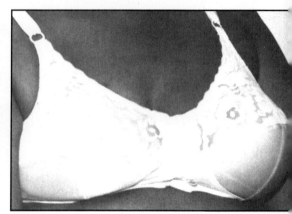

Figs. 12-8 / 12-9. Prosthesis, a small spongy cushion approximates the size of the remaining breast. It is placed in the bra to allow proper symmetry and fitting of clothes.

Occasionally the surgeon and patient desire nipple reconstruction in addition to providing the breast mound. In some early cancers the nipple of the diseased breast can be transplanted to another part of the body during mastectomy; and when breast reconstruction is carried out, the areola-nipple is simply placed in the appropriate location. If the original nipple can not be used then the plastic surgeon must reconstruct the areola-nipple complex derived from the labia adjacent to the vagina or from the opposite normal nipple.

Plastic surgeons at the Medical College of Virginia report using dermabrasion exclusively in black women to darken the skin and placing a small piece of plastic under the center to simulate a nipple.[5] Dermabrasion is the removal of the very top layer of skin. When it heals it leaves a darkened area. Then a small plastic chip is slid under the skin to the center of the darkened areola and an acceptable reconstructed nipple-areola is formed. This new procedure apparently is only applicable in black and other dark skinned women. Dermabrasion will not give a satisfactory darkening in fair-skinned women; but for black patients it is another tool available for the plastic surgeon.

Many women have found a waning enthusiasm for plastic surgery as they adjust during the first few months after mastectomy. When the reconstruction procedure and possible complications are fully explained, it

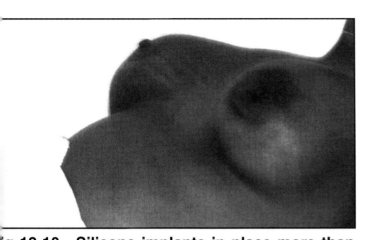

Fig 12-10. Silicone implants in place more than 5 years. There is leakage and chronic pain.

is not uncommon for the husband and the patient to indicate their preference for postponement.

On the other hand, many women desire reconstructive surgery or at least wish to know the possibilities available. Indeed these operations are getting better all the time and careful consideration with the plastic surgeon may be warranted. Be certain you understand what plastic surgery can and cannot do! Understand the risks and possible complications.

After silicone implant surgery an occasional patient will find their way back to the plastic surgeon to have their silicone implant removed. But removal is also mired in the backwater of controversy and complication. Removal of the implant may result in the nipple being much lower on the breast or hidden in the crease below the breast. The flabby, lax breast may require some sort of elevation or flap surgery to improve the general appearance. These procedures can be complicated by bleeding, infection, and delayed healing. One plastic surgeon may be reluctant to remove the implant knowing the possible complications and poor cosmetic outcome to be expected. Another plastic surgeon may be tempted to engage in a complicated endeavor of flaps and stents, with the expectation of financial reward.

In the coming years, I suspect, more women will be opting for lesser surgery, and preservation of the normal breast when the cancer is removed; and this will lessen the role of plastic surgery.

———

Along with the practical choices you must make about mastectomy, lumpectomy, plastic surgery, chemotherapy, radiation, Tamoxifen and other treatments, you've got to adopt the correct attitude and develop a positive point of view.

A personal physician or clinic can direct you to the right medical professionals that in turn will guide you through the first weeks of rehabilitation and decision making. That's fine. But you must come to grips with what is essential and important in your life. Only you can define what is important and what is superfluous.

It is time to boldly step up on the stage of life, back straight, head held high. It is still your show, you know. Family and friends may represent a major part of the supporting cast of players; but only *you* can make it work.

After taking care of the tangible choices that lend themselves to a "Things to Do" list, you've got to get into the realm of the psyche and the spirit. It is the mystical side of your being that sustains you—that sustains all of us. It's what makes a singer like Abby Lincoln go on stage in spite of fever and physical weakness. Strength comes from the spirit and the will. No one quite understands it. It is a mysterious presence. Perhaps we get a bit closer to a definition when we marvel at the nature and handiwork of God that we witness all around us everyday. Philosophers use parables and metaphors. Poets use rhyme and syntax. The preacher shouts from the pulpit; and we call on it through prayer and meditation. It is invisible, but real—impossible to describe. And yet it's that well that we must all tap to reap the fullness that life offers. I suppose it will always be a riddle. Like 'seeing through a glass darkly'. Some call it faith. 'The evidence of things not seen'. If you use it right it will sustain you and comfort you like a child knowing, 'Daddy won't let me fall'. Every week Dr Frederick KC Price declares from the Faithdome, "We walk by faith, not by sight!"

Personal tragedy must come to all; but when that intruder crosses your doorstep, embrace him with quiet equanimity. Like Fleetwood Mack sings "Don't stop—thinking about tomorrow! Yesterday's gone. Yesterday's gone."

It does not matter at what time your day begins or what the weather. If you awaken to sunshine and birds singing, or if you're shaken from a fitful slumber before dawn, and peer out the window at a driving rain, wind whistling through the trees, in either case simply exclaim, "Thank God for this beautiful day". Should the thunder crash loud, and electricity crack the somber sky—know that God's eyes are flashing, his voice is roaring, and the earth is trembling. We are being reminded that we are but filthy rags

Lights, Camera, Action!

before His Majesty. This is a time in life to awake in the morning simply thankful for another opportunity to do something positive, to make a difference, to find peace, perhaps to bring joy to somebody with a word or gesture.

This is a time in life for quiet reflection, for introspection. Look at the storm in your life, and run to the rock (I Corinthians 10:4). Remember these words, 'Be still and know that I am God'. We can only live one day at a time, so make this day, today, special! Greet each day with your personal agenda. Think of reasonable things that can be accomplished, and experience the contentment that comes with accomplishment regardless of how small.

In the final analysis this life is still your show and the show must go on! It remains for you, only you, to take the time to remember and savor the good things and the blessings you *have* received in spite of the present alarm and trepidation. In spite of it all, it is still you who must find the inner power and faith to go on. So study your lines and get ready for the rest of your life! Get up on that stage. Curtain's going up. Your audience awaits you. It's time for lights! It's time for camera! It is time for action!

"Education, income, and health insurance status are more important in determining the likelihood of receiving screening mammography than race" (according to Victor G Vogel, MD, - Director of The Breast Cancer Program at the University of Pittsburgh Cancer Institute). This may be true, but, tell me, who is most educationally deprived, who is disproportionately poor, and who is most likely to be without health insurance? Black folks! And guess who is less likely to have a mammogram. You!

APPENDIX A

National Breast Cancer Advocacy Organizations

The Office of Special Populations (The National Cancer Institute)
301 402 63

The American Cancer Society
3340 Peachtree Road NE
Atlanta, GA 30026
800 ACS 2345

The Susan G Komen Breast Cancer Foundation
Occidental Tower 5005 LBJ Freeway Suite 370 Dallas, TX 75244
800 462 9273

National Breast Cancer Coalition [NBCC]
1707 L Street NW Suite 1060 Washington, DC 20036
202 296 7477

Breast Cancer.net
732 224 0402

Avon Breast Cancer Awareness Crusade

Breast Cancer Information Clearing House
Accessible via the Internet http://nysernet.org/bcic/

Y-ME National Breast Cancer Organization
212 West Van Buren 5th Floor Chicago, IL 60607-3908
800 221 2141

National Alliance of Breast Cancer Organizations [NABCO]
9 East 37th Street 10th Floor New York NY 10016
800 719 9154

African American Breast Cancer Alliance [AABCA]
PO Box 88981, Minneapolis, MN 55435
612 825 3675 or 612 925 2772

Breast Cancer Resource Committee [BCRC]
1765 N Street NW Washington, DC 20036
202 463 8040

Circle of Friends
Women Telling Women About Breast anc Cervical Cancer
National Caucus and Center on Black Aged, Inc
1424 K Street NW Suite 500 Washington DC 20005
202 637 8400

The YWCA Encore Program
726 Broadway
New York,NY 10003
212 614 2827

APPENDIX B

African American Breast Cancer Support and Survivor Groups

SISTERS NETWORK--Chapter Locations:

TEXAS

National Headquarters
Karen Jackson, National President
8787 Woodway Drive #4207
Houston, TX 770 63
(713) 781 0255

Lois Williams, President
1610 Brandy Lane
Allen, TX 75002
(214) 637 7451

ALABAMA

Doris Epps, President
Chattahoochee Valley Chapter
8 Epps Crossing Road
Seale, AL 36875-4710

LOUISIANA

Gwendolyn D Brooks, President
Baton Rouge Chapter
7126 Dalark Drive
Baton Rouge, LA 70812-1313
(504) 355 2661

NEW YORK

Wilma Carroll, President
315 Lynn Court
Uniondale, NY 11533
(516) 538-8086

Maria Rankins, President
Sisters Network-Austin Chapt.
PO Box 151255
Austin, TX 78715-1255
(512) 422 8087

E Carolyn Beaman, President
123 Poinciana
Lake Jackson, TX 77566
(409) 297 4419

CALIFORNIA

Gloria Harmon, President
Women of Essence
PO Box 1854
Lynwood, CA 90262

MARYLAND

Jacqueline Chambers, Pres.
Sisters Surviving
16 Brickford Lane
Pikesville, MA 21208
(410) 486 6325

Margie L Bhola, President
Queens New York Chapter
PO Box 204
Brooklyn, NY 11207
(718) 723 5879 (fax) 723 5563

Other African American Support and Survivor Groups

Rise Sister Rise
1765 N Street NW
Washington DC 20036
Zora Kramer Brown, Founder
202 463 8040

Sisters Breast Cancer Survivors Network
YWCA Greater Los Angeles
2501 W Vernon Avenue
Los Angeles CA 90008
213 293 9408

Women of Color Breast Cancer Survivors Support Project
8610 S Sapulveda Suite 200
LosAngeles, CA 90045

Embracing Life
National Black Leadership Initiative on Cancer
University of Illinois at Chicago
2121 W Taylor Street Suite 512
Chicago IL 60612
312 996 8046

Beauty and the Breast
American Cancer Society
241 Fourth Avenue
Pittsburgh, PA 15222

APPENDIX C

States with Informed Consent Laws Regarding Breast Cancer Treatment

STATE	STATE LAW	INFO PROVIDED	CONSENT
California	Code 1704.5	Altern. Treatm.	Required
Florida	Statue 458.324	Altern. Treatm	Required
Georgia	Code 43-34-2	Altern. Treatm.	Required
Kentucky	Statue 311.935	Altern. Treatm.	Required
Maine	Satue 24.2905A	Altern. Treatm.	Required
Maryland	Law 20.113	Altern. Treatm.	Required
Mass.	Statue 111.70E	Altern. Treatm.	Required
Michigan	Statue 333.17013	Altern. Treatm.	Required
Minnesota	Statue 144.651	Altern. Treatm.	Required
New York	Law 2404	Altern. Treatm.	Required
Texas	Code 86.001	Altern. Treatm.	Required

APPENDIX D

Selected List of Breast Cancer Clinical Trials
[ongoing in 1997]

Adjuvant Tamoxifen Therapy and Ovarian Ablation in Node-Negative, Receptor-Positive Breast Cancer

This phase III trial studies the addition of ovarian ablation to Tamoxifen as an adjuvant treatment of women whose breast cancer on initial diagnosis tests estrogen receptor positive and/or progesterone-receptor positive, and who have negative axillary lymph nodes and a diagnosis of stage I or stage II breast cancer. Trial participants must be premenopausal, and begin the study within 12 weeks of their initial surgery for breast cancer. Patients will be randomized to one of two groups: those taking Tamoxifen by mouth for 5 years, or those who in addition to taking Tamoxifen for 5 years undergo ovarian ablation. The method of ovarian ablation can be selected by the patient and her physician, and may be by surgery, radiation therapy, or drug treatment. In addition to meeting the requirements described, eligible patients are those whose breast cancer is 3 centimeters or less in diameter and have no other serious medical problems. For more information, call Dr. Nicholas Robert at 703-698-3653, Dr. Richard Schilsky at 312-702-6180, Dr. James Ingle at 507-284-2511, or Dr. Silvana Martino at 805-446-4950.

Adjuvant Hormonal Therapy in Node-Positive, Receptor-Positive Breast Cancer

This phase III trial studies the addition of fenretinide to Tamoxifen as an adjuvant treatment for women whose breast cancer on initial diagnosis tests estrogen receptor positive or progesterone-receptor positive and who have positive axillary lymph nodes -- a diagnosis of stage II or stage III breast cancer. Trial participants must be postmenopausal, and begin the study within 12 weeks of their initial surgery for breast cancer. Patients will be randomized to one of two groups: those taking Tamoxifen plus fenretinide, or those taking Tamoxifen plus a placebo, by mouth once a day for 5 years. In addition to meeting the requirements described, eligible patients are those with no previous breast cancer treatment other than surgery; who have refused treatment in certain other trials and have no other serious medical problems or problems with vision. For more information, call Dr. Melody Cobleigh at 312-942-3240, Dr. Mark Graham at 919-966-4431, or

Dr. James Ingle at 507-284-2511.

Radiation Therapy and Tamoxifen in Very Early Stage Node-Negative Invasive Breast Cancer

This phase III trial compares radiation therapy plus Tamoxifen, radiation therapy plus placebo, and Tamoxifen alone as adjuvant therapy for breast cancer. Patients randomized to the first two groups will receive radiation therapy to the breast and take either a placebo or Tamoxifen by mouth twice each day for 5 years. Patients randomized to the third group will not receive radiation therapy, but will take Tamoxifen twice each day for 5 years. Eligible patients are those with newly diagnosed invasive breast cancer that is 1 centimeter or less in size, who have negative axillary lymph nodes and have no other serious medical problems. For more information, call Dr. Norman Wolmark at 412-359-3336, Dr. Robert Carlson at 415-723-7621, or Dr. James Ahlgren at 202-994-2746.

Immunotherapy after Surgery for Breast Cancer

The purpose of this phase III trial is to study adjuvant therapy with Corynebacterium granulosum following surgery for breast cancer. Beginning 2 weeks after surgery, patients will receive life-long therapy consisting of injections once a week for 6 weeks followed by a 3-month rest. To be eligible, patients must be 20-80 years old and have had surgery that removed at least 90% of their tumor. For more information, call Hugo Omar De Carli at 021-84-3119.

Adjuvant Tamoxifen for Breast Cancer in Patients Older Than 50 Years

The purpose of this phase III trial is to compare 2 years versus 5 years of Tamoxifen adjuvant therapy in women older than 50 years with stage I breast cancer or stage II breast cancer. All patients will receive 2 years of Tamoxifen daily by mouth beginning as soon after surgery as possible. Patients will then be randomized to one of two groups: those who receive 3 more years of Tamoxifen or those who receive no further therapy. Physicians may also choose to randomize patients to receive radiation therapy and/or CMF chemotherapy or may designate certain groups of patients to these treatments. To be eligible, patients must be between 50 and 74 years old and have no other serious medical problems.

Surgery plus Radiation Therapy for Paget's Disease of the Nipple Associated with Ductal Carcinoma In Situ

The purpose of this phase II trial is to study the surgical removal of

Paget's disease of the nipple, followed by radiation therapy in patients who have ductal carcinoma in situ. All patients will undergo removal of the cancer within 6 weeks after biopsy. Radiation therapy will be given for 5 weeks, beginning 1 to 3 weeks after surgery. To be eligible, patients must be younger than 70 years old and must not have previously received any other anti-cancer therapy. For more information, call Emile J. Rutgers at 31-20-512-9111

Adjuvant Hormone Therapy for Operable Breast Cancer

The purpose of this phase III trial is to study the use of Tamoxifen, ovarian ablation, or both as adjuvant therapy for women with stage I breast cancer or stage II breast cancer. All patients will undergo surgery and may receive chemotherapy cyclophosphamide, or radiation therapy. Patients will be randomized to one of four groups for at least 2 years of adjuvant treatment: those who receive no further treatment, those who receive Tamoxifen alone, those who receive goserelin alone, and those who receive both Tamoxifen and goserelin. To be eligible, patients must be younger than 50 years old and have no other serious medical problems. For more information, call Michael Baum at 171 380-9147

Radiation Therapy and Tamoxifen in Very Early Stage Breast Cancer

The purpose of this phase III trial is to compare radiation therapy plus tamoxifen, radiation therapy plus placebo, and tamoxifen alone in women with stage I breast cancer. Patients will be randomized to one of three groups. The first group will receive radiation therapy to the breast plus tamoxifen every day for 5 years. The second group will receive radiation therapy to the breast plus placebo every day for 5 years. The third group will receive only Tamoxifen every day for 5 years. To be eligible, patients must be within 9 weeks of their initial diagnosis and their tumors must have been 1 centimeter or less in size and have been removed by breast-conserving surgery. For more information, call Norman Wolmark at 412-359-3336, Robert W. Carlson at 415-723-7621 or James D. Ahlgren at 202-994-2746

Neoadjuvant versus Adjuvant Combination Chemotherapy in Women with Stage II Breast Cancer

The purpose of this phase III trial is to study combination chemotherapy as either neoadjuvant therapy or adjuvant therapy in women with stage II breast cancer. Patients will be randomized to receive fluorouracil, leucovorin, doxorubicin, clophosphamide, and G-CSF for 15 weeks either before or after surgery. Some patients will also receive radiation therapy for up to 7.5 weeks after completion of surgery and chemotherapy. In addition to the requirements above, patients must be 20 to 70 years old and must have no other serious medical problems. Patients with bilateral breast cancer are eligible provided neither tumor is stage III breast cancer. For more information, call David N. Danforth, Jr. at 301-496-1533

Adjuvant Therapy in Premenopausal and Perimenopausal Women with Node-Negative Breast Cancer
The purpose of this phase III trial is to compare adjuvant therapy with goserelin alone, CMF alone, or CMF followed by goserelin in premenopausal and perimenopausal women with stage I breast cancer or stage II breast cancer with negative axillary lymph nodes who have had the cancer removed by surgery. Patients must begin treatment within 6 weeks of surgery. Patients will be randomized to one of four groups: those who receive no further therapy, those who receive goserelin monthly for 2 years, those who receive CMF monthly for 6 months, or those who receive CMF for 6 months followed by goserelin monthly for 18 months. Patients who did not have a mastectomy may choose to also receive radiation therapy. To be eligible, patients must have had axillary lymph nodes removed at surgery, have cancer in only one breast, and have no other serious medical problems. In addition, patients should not have received any prior chemotherapy, radiation therapy, or biologic or hormone therapy for breast cancer. For more information, call Monica Castiglione-Gertsch at 011-41-31-389-9191

Conventional versus Intensive Adjuvant Combination Chemotherapy, with versus without Hormone Therapy, for Poor Risk Breast Cancer
The purpose of this phase III trial is to compare adjuvant therapy with either AC or CMF plus either Tamoxifen or placebo in women with stage I or stage II breast cancer that is estrogen receptor negative. Patients must be randomized to one of four groups within 5 weeks of surgery. Two groups will receive CMF for 6 months and either tamoxifen or placebo by mouth daily for 5 years; the other two groups will receive AC for 12 weeks and either tamoxifen or placebo by mouth daily for 5 years. Radiation therapy is given after the first month of CMF therapy and after completion of AC therapy. To be eligible, patients must be between 18 and 75 years old, have a tumor at least 1 centimeter in size, and have no other serious medical problems. For more information, call Norman Wolmark at 412-359-3336

Tamoxifen versus No Further Treatment Following Adjuvant Chemotherapy for Stage I/II Breast Cancer

The purpose of this phase III trial is to study tamoxifen following adjuvant therapy in the treatment of women with stage I breast cancer or stage II breast cancer. Patients will be randomized to one of two groups within 2 weeks of completing adjuvant chemotherapy: those who receive tamoxifen daily by mouth for 3 years or those who receive no further treatment. To be eligible, patients must have received at least six courses of prior adjuvant chemotherapy with one of five specified regimens, have had the cancer completely removed by surgery, and have had a mammogram within 1 year of entry showing no cancer in the opposite breast. For more information, call Peter F. Bruning at 011-31-20-512-2569

Breast Surgery with or without Lymph Node Removal in Elderly Women

The purpose of this phase III trial is to study the extent of surgery that should be used in women older than 70 years old who have stage I breast cancer or stage II breast cancer with no known positive axillary lymph nodes. Patients will be randomized to one of two groups: those who undergo breast surgery with removal of axillary lymph nodes or those who undergo breast surgery without removal of axillary lymph nodes. Following surgery, both groups receive adjuvant therapy with tamoxifen daily by mouth for 5 years. Patients who underwent breast-conserving surgery may also receive radiation therapy. To be eligible, patients must have cancer in only one breast, have received no previous breast cancer therapy except biopsy of the breast, and have no other serious medical problems. For more information, call Diana Crivellari at 39-434-659206

Hormone Therapy with or without Chemotherapy for Node-Positive Breast Cancer

The purpose of this phase III trial is to compare hormone therapy alone with hormone therapy plus chemotherapy as adjuvant therapy in premenopausal women with positive axillary lymph nodes. All patients will undergo ovarian ablation. They will then be randomized to one of two groups: those receiving tamoxifen by mouth daily for 5 years or those receiving cyclophosphamide with either epirubicin or doxorubicin monthly for 4 months followed by Tamoxifen daily by mouth for 5 years. To be eligible, patients must be younger than 50 years old, have cancer in only one breast, have completed surgery, and have no other serious medical problems. For more information, call Beat Thurlimann at 071-494-1067

Effect of Treatment Delay on Adjuvant Regimens in Premenopausal

Women with Node-Positive Breast Cancer

The purpose of this phase III trial is to examine a rest between adjuvant therapy with two chemotherapy regimens with or without Tamoxifen for the treatment of premenopausal women with stage II breast cancer with positive axillary lymph nodes or stage III A breast cancer. Patients will be randomized to one of four groups: 1) for 12 weeks followed immediately by CMF for 12 weeks; 2) AC and CMF as in group 1, but separated by 16 weeks; 3) AC and CMF as in group 1, followed by tamoxifen daily by mouth for 4.5 years; and 4) AC and CMF as group 2, with tamoxifen daily by mouth for 4.5 years. Some patients will also receive radiation therapy. To be eligible, patients must have cancer in only one breast, have received no previous breast cancer therapy other than surgery, and have no other serious medical problems. For more information, call Alan Stuart Coates at 612-9515-6123

Effect of Treatment Delay on Adjuvant Regimens in Perimenopausal and Postmenopausal Women with Node-Positive Breast Cancer

The purpose of this phase III trial is to examine a rest between adjuvant therapy with two chemotherapy regimens with either tamoxifen or to remifene for the treatment of perimenopausal or postmenopausal women with stage II breast cancer with positive axillary lymph nodes or stage IIIA breast cancer who are not candidates for hormone therapy alone. Patients will be randomized to one of four groups: 1) AC for 12 weeks followed immediately by CMF for 12 weeks, followed by Tamoxifen daily by mouth for 4.5 years; 2) AC and CMF separated by 16 weeks of rest, then followed by Tamoxifen daily by mouth for 4.25 years; 3) AC and CMF as in group 1, followed by toremifene daily by mouth for 4.5 years; and 4) AC and CMF as in group 2, followed by toremifene daily by mouth for 4.25 years. Some patients will also receive radiation therapy. To be eligible, patients must be younger than 70 years old, have cancer in only one breast, have received no previous breast cancer therapy other than surgery, and have no other serious medical problems. For more information, call Dr. Pagani at 0041-92-269147

Adjuvant Therapy in Node-Negative Breast Cancer

The purpose of this phase III trial is to compare no adjuvant therapy, radiation therapy alone, Tamoxifen alone, and radiation therapy plus Tamoxifen in women with stage I breast cancer who have undergone surgery for tumor removal. Patients will be randomized to one of four groups: 1)those observed without treatment, 2) those who receive radiation therapy to the breast for 5-6 weeks, 3) those who receive Tamoxifen by mouth daily for 5 years, or 4) those who receive both radiation therapy for 5-6 weeks plus Tamoxifen by mouth daily for 5 years. To be eligible, patients must be between 45 and 75 years old, have estrogen or progesterone receptor positive breast cancer, and have no other serious medical problems. For more information, call Helmut F. Rauschecker at 09131-853404

Tamoxifen with or without Radiation Therapy for Node-negative Breast Cancer in Elderly Women

The purpose of this phase III trial is to study the addition of radiation therapy to Tamoxifen following breast-conserving surgery in patients with stage I or stage II breast cancer with negative axillary lymph nodes. Patients must be over 70 years old and begin therapy within 12 weeks of surgery. All patients will receive Tamoxifen daily by mouth for 5 years. Patients will be randomized to one of two groups: those who receive radiation therapy over 6 weeks when they begin taking Tamoxifen; or those who receive no therapy in addition to Tamoxifen. To be eligibl e, patients must have had a tumor that was no larger than 2 cm. Any estrogen replacement therapy must be discontinued prior to entry. For more information, call Kevin S. Hughes at 617-273-8573 or Thomas Julius Smith at 201-971-5678

Adjuvant Tamoxifen Following CMF in Women with Operable Invasive Breast Cancer

The purpose of this phase III trial is to study adjuvant therapy with Tamoxifen following CMF in women with stage I or stage II breast cancer that can be removed by surgery. Within 4 weeks after surgery, all patients will receive CMF every 3 weeks for 18 weeks. Before completion of CMF, patients will be randomized to one of two groups: those who receive Tamoxifen daily by mouth for 5 years or those who receive no additional therapy. Some patients will receive radiation therapy. Women may be either premenopausal or postmenopausal, must not have received Tamoxifen previously, and must have no other serious health problems. For more information, call W.D. George at 0141-211-2166

Adjuvant Tamoxifen, Ovarian Ablation, and CMF in Premenopausal Women with Operable Invasive Breast Cancer

The purpose of this phase III trial is to study adjuvant therapy with various combinations of Tamoxifen, ovarian ablation, and in premenopausal women with stage I or stage II breast cancer that can be removed by surgery. Within 2 weeks after surgery, patients will be randomized to one of four groups: one group receives Tamoxifen daily by mouth for 5 years; the second group receives Tamoxifen daily by mouth for 5 years plus CMF every 3 weeks for 18 weeks; the third group receives Tamoxifen daily by mouth for 5 years plus ovarian ablation by surgery, radiation therapy, or hormone therapy; and the fourth group receives treatment with Tamoxifen daily by mouth for 5 years plus CMF every 3 weeks for 18 weeks and undergoes ovarian ablation. Treatment must begin within 4 weeks of surgery. Some patients will also receive additional radiation therapy. To be eligible, women must have no other serious health problems. For more information, call W.D. George at 0141-211-2166

Adjuvant Tamoxifen Alone or with CMF in Postmenopausal Women with Operable Invasive Breast Cancer

The purpose of this phase III trial is to study adjuvant therapy with Tamoxifen alone or with CMF in postmenopausal women with stage I or stage II breast cancer that can be removed by surgery. Within 2 weeks after surgery, patients will be randomized to one of two groups: those who receive Tamoxifen by mouth for 5 years or those who receive Tamoxifen plus CMF every 3 weeks for 18 weeks. Treatment must begin within 4 weeks of surgery. Selected patients will also receive radiation therapy. Eligible women must have no other serious health problems. For more information, call W.D. George at 0141-211-2166 The PDQ summary contains a detailed, more technical trial description and list of the physicians participating in this trial.

Adjuvant Tamoxifen, Ovarian Suppression, and/or Chemotherapy for Early Stage Breast Cancer

The purpose of this phase III trial is to study the survival of women with stage I or stage II and some women with stage IIIA breast cancer who receive adjuvant therapy with Tamoxifen, chemotherapy, and/or ovarian ablation. Patients will be randomized to one of four treatment groups: one group receives Tamoxifen alone daily by mouth for 5 years; the second group receives Tamoxifen daily by mouth for 5 years plus combination chemotherapy with either for 6 months or doxorubicin and cyclophosphamide for 3 months; a third group receives Tamoxifen daily by mouth for 5 years plus either removal of the ovaries by surgery or suppression of ovarian function by radiation therapy or by leuprolide or goserelin; and a fourth group receives Tamoxifen daily by mouth for 5 years plus chemotherapy plus ovarian suppression. Patients must have had no previous treatment for breast cancer. For more information, call John Robert Arnold at 081-642-6011, Stanley Bernard Kaye at 0141-221-2824, Murray Brunt at 01782-716588, Tim Perren at 113 283 70 35 or Helena Earl at

021-414-3787

Adjuvant Tamoxifen and Ovarian Ablation in Node-Negative, Receptor-Positive Breast Cancer

The purpose of this phase III trial is to study the addition of ovarian ablation to Tamoxifen as an adjuvant therapy for women with stage I or stage II breast cancer that is estrogen and/or progesterone receptor positive and who have negative axillary lymph nodes. Patients must be and begin the study within 12 weeks of their initial surgery for breast cancer. Patients will be randomized to one of two groups: those who take Tamoxifen by mouth daily for 5 years or those who take Tamoxifen for 5 years and undergo ovarian ablation. The method of ovarian ablation can be selected by the patient and her physician and may be by surgery, radiation therapy, or drug treatment. In addition to the above requirements, eligible participants must have breast cancer that is less than 3 centimeters in diameter and have no other serious medical problems. For more information, call Nicholas J. Robert at 703-698-3653, Debasish Tripathy at 415-502-0873, James N. Ingle at 507-284-2511 or Silvana Martino at 805-446-4950

Adjuvant Hormone Therapy with or without CMF in Postmenopausal Women with Node-Negative Breast Cancer

The purpose of this phase III trial is to study combination chemotherapy followed by Tamoxifen versus Tamoxifen alone in postmenopausal women with stage I or stage II breast cancer with negative axillary lymph nodes. Patients will be randomized to one of two groups: those who receive Tamoxifen daily by mouth for 5 years or those who receive CMF monthly for 3 months followed by Tamoxifen daily by mouth for 5 years. Radiation therapy to the breast will be optional for those who underwent breast-conserving surgery. To be eligible, patients must be older than 16 years, have cancer in only one breast, have had no previous treatment for breast cancer other than surgery, and have no other serious medical problems. For more information, call Monica Castiglione-Gertsch at 011-41-31-389-9191

Radiation Therapy Following Surgery for Stage I Breast Cancer

The purpose of this phase III trial is to study adjuvant therapy with radiation therapy following breast-conserving surgery in women with stage I breast cancer at low risk for recurrence. Patients will be to one of two groups: those who receive 5 weeks of radiation therapy, beginning within 6 weeks after surgery; or those who receive no radiation therapy. Tamoxifen daily by mouth for a total of 3 years is allowed for all patients.

Trial participants must be at least 50 years old, have cancer in only one breast, not have Paget's disease of the nipple, and not have received other adjuvant therapy except Tamoxifen. For more information, call Mugginess Blichert-Toft at 45-35452117 or Harry Bartelink at 31-20-5122122

Docetaxel Before or After Surgery or No Docetaxel for Women with Operable Breast Cancer

The purpose of this phase III trial is to study the addition of docetaxel to adjuvant therapy with doxorubicin and cyclophosphamide (AC)in women with stage II or stage III breast cancer. All patients will receive AC over 3 months, then undergo surgery to remove their cancer; some patients will receive radiation therapy. All patients will receive Tamoxifen by mouth daily for 5 years. Patients will be randomized to receive docetaxel in one of three groups: those who receive it with AC prior to surgery, those who receive it after recovery from surgery, or those who receive no docetaxel. To be eligible, patients must have had no previous therapy for breast cancer, be free of serious cardiac disease, and not take oral contraceptives or estrogen replacement therapy while on study. For more information, call Harry D. Bear at 804-828-9325

Surgery with or without Lymph Node Removal in Elderly Women with Stage I Breast Cancer

The purpose of this phase III trial is to study the addition of axillary lymph node dissection to quadrantectomy in women with stage I breast cancer that is estrogen receptor positive. Patients will be to one of two groups: those who receive quadrantectomy with lymph node dissection or those who receive quadrantectomy alone. All patients receive Tamoxifen by mouth once a day for 5 years. To be eligible, women must be between 65 and 80 years old and have no medical problems that make them ineligible for surgery. For more information, call Gabriele Martelli at 39-2-2390-324

Standard versus Shortened Radiation Therapy for Node-Negative Breast Cancer

The purpose of this phase III trial is to compare standard radiation therapy with a higher dose and shorter course of radiation therapy as adjuvant therapy following lumpectomy in women with stage I and stage II breast cancer with negative axillary lymph nodes. Therapy must begin within 16 weeks after surgery (or 8 weeks after the completion of adjuvant chemotherapy, when given). Patients will be randomized to one of two groups: those who receive standard doses of radiation therapy over 35 days or those who receive higher doses of radiation therapy over 23 days. To be eligible, patients must have a tumor smaller than 5 cm, cancer in only one breast, and no other serious medical problems. For more information, call Drew C.G. Bethune at 902-428-4200.

Appendix D

REFERENCES

CHAPTER 1

1.Incidence of breast cancer (response to letter).JNCI 80:2, 1988

2. Kern KA: Causes of Breast Cancer Malpractice Litigation: A 20-year civil court review. Arch Surg 127:542-547, 1992

3. Bagle J Burnette C: The effects of breast cancer disclosure legislation on physician disclosure practices [dissertation]. Baltimore, The Johns Hopkins University, 1989

CHAPTER 3

1. Strax P: Advances in detection of early breast cancer; Cancer detection and prevention. 6:409-414 1983 pub. Alan R Liss Inc

2. Young JL Devesa SS Cutler SJ: Incidence of cancer in United States Blacks. Cancer Research 35:3523-3536 Nov 1975

3. Foster RS Costanza MC: Breast self-examination practices and breast cancer survival. Cancer 53:4 999-1005 Feb 15 1984

4. Lesnick GL: How best to proceed when the diagnosis is 'fibrocystic breast disease'. Your Patient and Cancer Feb 1983

5. Greenblatt RB Nexhat C Ben-Hur J: Treatment of benign breast disease with danazol. Fertil Steril 34:242 1980

6. Goldenburg IS Gump FE Minton JP et al: When breasts are fibrocystic. Patient Care 16:103-107 March 1982

7. Black MM Barclay THC Cutler SJ Hankey BF et al: Association of atypical characteristics of benign breast lesions with subsequent risk of breast cancer. Cancer 29:338-343 1972

8. Devitt JE: Breast cancer and preceding clinical benign breast disorders- a chance association. Lancet 793-795 April 10, 1976

9. Groveman HD Norcross WA: Adolescent breast masses. Hospital Medicine 65-84 May 1982

10. Lester RG: Risk versus benefit in mammography. Radiology 124:1 1977

11. Shapiro S Strax P Venet L: Periodic breast cancer screening in reducing mortality from breast cancer. JAMA 215: 1777-1785 1971

12. Wolf JN: Risk for breast cancer development determined by mammographic parenchymal pattern. Cancer 37:2486 1976

13. Krook PM Carlile T Bush W et al: Mammographic parenchymal patterns as a risk indicator for prevalent and incident cancer. Cancer 41:1093-1097 1978

14. Gautherie M Gross CM: Breast thermography and cancer risk prediction. Cancer 45:51-56 Jan 1980

15. Teixidor HS Elias K: Combined mammographic-sonographic evaluation of the breast. March 1977

16. Toomes H Vogt-Moykopf I: Surgery advised for palliative treatment of lung metastases. Reported at 14th annual Congress on Diseases of the Chest (American College of Chest Physicians). Family Practice News 13:3 Feb 1-14 1983 pp 85

17. Fisher E Sass R Fisher B: Biological considerations regarding the one and two step procedures in the management of patients with invasive carcinoma of the breast. SG&O 161:245-249 September 1985

18. Lee YTW: CEA in patients with breast...cancer; West J Med 129:374-380 Nov 1978

19. Tormey DC Walkes TP Snyder JJ Simon RM: Biological markers in breast carcinoma. III. Clinical correlations with carcinoembryonic antigen. Cancer 1977 Jun;(6) :2397-2404

20. Olszewski W Zbigniew D Rosen PP et al: Flow Cytometry of breast carcinoma: I. Relation of DNA Plody Level to histology and estrogen receptor. Cancer 48:4 Aug 15 1981 980-988

21. "Value of mammograms in younger women questioned": Amer Med News page 3; March 22/29 1993

22. Holzel WG Beer R Descher W et al: Individual reference ranges of CA 15-3, MCA and CEA in recurrence of breast cancer;Scand J Clin Lab Invest Suppl;221:93-101 1995

23. Jager W Kramer S Palapelas V Norbert L: Breast cancer and clinical utility of CA 15-3 and CEA; Scand J Clin Lab Invest Suppl 21:87-92 1995

24. Coveney EC Geraghty JG Sherry F et al: The clinical value of CEA and CA 15-3 in breast cancer management;Int J Biol Markers : 10(1) :35-41 Jan -Mar 1995

25. Giai M Yu H Roagna R et al: Prostatic-specific antigen in serum of women with breast cancer; Br J Canc 72(3):728-31 Sep 1995

26. Parker SL Tong T Bolden S Wingo PA: Cancer statistics, 1996;CA-A Can Jour for Clinicians 46:1 Jan Feb p 8 1996

27. Bird RE: Professional quality assurance for mammography screening programs; Radio 1177:587 1990

28. Tabar L Fagerberg G Duffy SW et al: Update of the Swedish two county program of mammographic screening for breast cancer Radiol Clin of N Amer 30:187-210 1992

29. Alcorn FS. Breast cancer detection: Mammography and other methods in breast imaging. second edition. Bassett LW Gold RH eds. Orlando Grune and Stratton, p 179-97, 1987)

30. Gemson DH Elinson J Messeri: Difference in physician prevention practice patterns for white and minority patients;J Comm Health 1988 Spring;13(1):53-64

31. Amir H Kwesigabo G Aziz M et al: Breast cancer and conservative surgery in sub saharan africa. East Afr Med J 1996 Feb;73(2):83-87

32. Bassett MT Levy L Chokunonga E et al: Cancer in the european population of harare, zimbabwe, 1990-192. Int J Cancer 1995 Sep 27;63(1):24-28

33. Elledge RM Clark GM Chamness GC Osborne CK: Tumor biologic factors and breast cancer prognosis among white, hispanic, and black women in the United States. J Nat Can Inst 1994 May 4; 86(9):705-712

34. Landercasper J Gundersen SB Gundersen AL et al: Needle localization and biopsy of nonpalpable lesions of the breast. SG&O 164:388-403, 1987

35. Shiao Y-H Chen VW Lehmann HP et al: Patterns of dna ploidy and s-phase fraction associated with breast cancer survival in blacks and whites.Clin Can Res 3:587-592 1997

CHAPTER 4

1. National Cancer Institute SEER Program 1973-1985

2. National Cancer Institute SEER Program 1973-1981

3. Young JL Devesa SS Cutler SJ: Incidence of Cancer in united states blacks. Cancer Research 35:Nov 1975 3523-3536

4. MacMahon, Cole P, Brown J: Etiology of human breast cancer: a review. J Natl Cancer Inst 50:21-42 1973

5. Anderson DE: Genetic study of breast cancer: identification of a high risk group. Cancer 34:1090-1097, 1974

6. Robbins G Berg JW: Bilateral primary breast cancer; a prospective clinical pathological study. Cancer 17:1501-1527, 1964

7. MacMahon B Cole P Lin TM et al: Age at first birth and breast cancer risk. Bull WHO 43:2909-221, 1970

8. Kamoi M: Statistical study on relation between breast cancer and lactation period. I. A comparative study through cumulative frequency distribution. Tohoku J Exp Med 72: 59-65 1960

9. Brody H Cullem M: Carcinoma of breast seventeen years after mammography with thorotrast. Surgery 42:600-606 1957

10. MacKenzie I: Breast cancer following multiple fluoroscopies. Brit J Cancer 19: 1-8, 165

11. Wanebo CK Johnson KG Sato K Thorslund TW: Breast cancer after exposure to the atomic bombing of hiroshima and nagasaki. NEJM 279:13 Sept 26, 1968 667-671

12. Warren S: The relation of "chronic mastitis" to carcinoma of the breast. SG&O 71:257-278, 1940

13. Black MM Barclay TH Cutler SJ et al: Association of atypical characteristic of benign breast lesions with subsequent risk of breast cancer. Cancer 29:338-343, 1972

14. Lemon HM: Abnormal estrogen metabolism and tissue estrogen receptor proteins in breast cancer. Cancer 25:423-435, 1970

15. Macdonald EJ: Ethnic and Regional Considerations in Epidemiology of breast cancer. J Amer Med Women's Asso 30:3 March 1975

16. Mirra AP Cole P MacMahon B: Breast cancer in an area of high parity; Sao Paulo Brazil. Cancer res.31:77, 1971

17. Lemon HM: Pathophysiologic considerations in the treatment of menopausal patients with estrogens; the role of estriol in the prevention of mammary carcinoma. Acta Endocrinologica 1980 Suppl.233: 17-27

18. Lipsett MB: Hormones, nutrition, and cancer. Cancer Research 35:3359-3361 Nov 1975

19. Henderson BE Gerkins V Rosario I et al: Elevated serum levels of estrogen and prolactin in daughters of patients with breast cancer. NEJM 293:16 790-794 Oct 16 1975

20. Hoover R Gray LA Cole P et al: Menopausal estrogens and breast cancer NEJM 295:8 401-405 Aug 19 1976

21. Fasal E Paffenbarger RS: Oral Contraceptives as related to cancer and benign lesions of the breast. J Nat. Cancer Inst 55:4 767-773 Oct 1975

22. Child M Vellios F Meigs JW et al: MMWR 31:29 393-394 July 30, 1982

23. Kapdi CC Wolfe JN: Breast cancer relationship to thyroid supplements for hypothyroidism JAMA 236:10 1124-1127 Sept 6, 1976

24. Lipsett MB: Hormones, nutrition, and cancer. Cancer Research 35: 3359-3361

25. deWaard F: Breast cancer incidence and nutritional status with particular reference to body weight and height. Cancer Research 35:3351-3356 Nov1975

26. Dickinson LE MacMahon B Cole P et al: Estrogen Profiles of oriental and caucasian women in hawaii NEJM 291:23 1211-1214 Dec 5, 1974

27. Carroll KK: Experimental evidence of dietary factors and hormone-dependent cancers. Cancer Research35:3374-3383 Nov 1975

28. Schechter MT Miller AB Howe GR et al: Cigarette smoking and breast cancer: case control studies of prevalent and incident cancer in the Canadian National Breast Screening Study. Am J Epidemiol 1989 Aug;130(2):213-220

29. Reed TE: Caucasian genes in american negroes. Science 165:762-768 Aug 22, 1969

30. Petrakis N: Some preliminary observations on the influence of genetic admixture on cancer incidence in american negroes. Int J Cancer 7:256-258 1971

31. American Cancer Society: Special Report on Cancer in the Economically disadvantaged, prepared by the Amer Can Soc, Sub comm on Can in the Economically Disadvantaged. New York, Amer Can Society,

1986

32. Bain RP Greenberg RS Whitaker JP: Racial differences in survival of women with breast cancer. J Chronic Dis 39:631-642, 1986

33. Ragland KE Selvin S Merrill DW: Black-white differences in stage specific cancer survival: Analysis of seven selected sites. Am J Epdemiol 133:672-682, 1991

34. Wynder EL MacCornack FA Stellman SD: The epidemology of breast cancer in 785 united states caucasian women. Cancer 41:6 June 1978 2341-2353

35. McWhorter WP Mayer WJ: Blac/white differences in type of initial breast cancer treatment and implications for survival. Am J Public Health 1987 Dec ;77 (12):1515-7

36. Mayer WJ McWhorter WP: Black/white differences in non-treatment of bladder cancer patients and implications for survival. Am J Public Health 1989 Jun;79(6):772-5

37. Coates RJ Bransfield DD Wesley M et al: Differences between black and white women with breast cancer in time from symptom recognition to medical consultation. Black/White survival study group. J Natl Cancer Inst (1992 Jun 17) 84(12):938-50

38. Garfinkel L: Current Trends in Breast Cancer. CA-A Can. J Phys.43:1 Jan/Feb 1993 pp 5-6.

39. Olsson H Moller TR Ranstam J: Early oral contraceptive use and breast cancer among premenopausal women: Final report from a study in southern Sweden. J Natl Cancer 1989;8

40. McDivitt RW Stevens JA Lee NC et al: Cancer and steroid hormone study group....Cancer 1992; 69:1408-14

41. White E: Rising incidence of breast cancer (response to letter).JNCI 80:2, 1988

42. Muss HB Hunter CP Wesley M et al: Treatment Plans for Black and White Women......: Cancer 70:2460-2467, 1992

Breast Cancer / Black Woman

43. Williams R Laing AE Demenais F et al: Descriptive analysis of breast cancer in african-american women at howard university hospital, 1960-1987;JNMA 85:11 828-34 Nov 1993

44. Bhatias S et al: Breast cancer and other second neoplasms after childhood Hodgkin's's disease; NEJM 334:745-51 Mar 21 1996

45 Donaldson SS Hancock SL: Second cancers after Hodgkin's disease in childhood;NEJM 334;792-94 Mar21 1996

46. Giani C et al: Relationship between breast cancer and thyroid disease: relevance of autoimmune thyroid disorders in breast malignancy. J Clin Endo Metab 81:990-94 Mar 1996

47. Laing AE Demenais FM Williams R et al: Breast cancer risk factors in african-american women:the howard university tumor registry experience;JNMA 85:12 931-39 Dec 1993

48. Daling JR Malone KE Voigt LF et al: Risk of breast cancer among young women. J Natl Can Inst 86:21 1584-92 Nov 2 1994

49. Cancer Statistics 1994: CA A Can J for Clin 45:1 Jan/Feb1995 p 27

50. Haabel LA Stanford JL et al: Occupation and breast cancer risk in middle-aged women. J Occup Environ Med 1995 Mar;37(3):349-56

51. Krieger N Wolff MS et al: Breast cancer and serum organochlorines: a prospective study among white, black, and Asian women. J Nat Can Inst 1994 Apr 20;86(8):589-99

52. Hancock SL et al: Breast cancer after treatment of hodgkin's disease. J Nat Can Inst Jan 6, 1993 p. 25-31

53. Coogan P: Electromagnetic fields and breast cancer. Epidemiol. 1996;457-64

54. Estrogen Users Get Receptor-Positive Breast Ca;Fam Prac News March 1, 1996 p.29

55. Bennicke et al: Effect of cigarette smoking on risk of breast

cancer;BMJ;310:June 3 1995

56. Nirmul D Pegoraro RJ Jialal I Naidoo C Thin IS Najem R Paradiso J Fuerman M: The sex hormone profile of male patients with breast cancer.BrJ Cancer 1983 Sep;48 (3):423-7

57. Kumar NB: Progressive weight gain increases risk of breast cancer.Cancer 1995;76:243-49

58. American Cancer Society. Cancer facts and figures 1996. Atlanta, Georgia: American Cancer Society, 1996; publication no. 5008.96

59. Kosary CL Ries LAG Miller Ba et al: eds. SEER cancer statistics review, 1973-92: tables and graphs. Bethesda, MD: Us Department of Health and Hu man Services, Public Gealth Service, National Institutes of Health, National Cancer Institute, 1995; publication no. (NIH)96- 2789

60. Whelan SL Parkin DM Masuyer R: World Health Organization Pattens of cancer in five continents;Lyo, France: International Agency for Research on Cancer, 1990.(IARC scientific publications no. 102)

61. Ambrosone CB Freudenheim JL Graham S et al: Cigarette smoking, n-acetyltransferase 2 genetic polymorphisms, and breast cancer risk;276:18 JAMA Nov 13, 1996

62. Hancock SL: Breast cancer after treatment of hodgkin's disease;JNCI Jan 6, 1993 25-31

63. Isaacs JH: Cancer of the breast in pregnancy; Surg Clin N Amer 75:47-51 1995

64. Holmes FA: Breast cancer during pregnancy; Cancer Bull 46;400-11 1994

65. Sutton NR Buzdar AU Hortobagyi GN: Pregnancy and offspring after adjuvant chemotherapy in breast cancer patients; Cancer 65:847-850 1990

66. Danforth DN Jr.: How subsequent pregnancy affects outcome in women with a prior breast cancer; Oncology 5:21-30 1991

67. Gerber M et al: Cancer Investigation 1991;9:421-8

68. Hoffer A: J Orthomolecular Med 3rd Quart. 1993;8:157-67

69. El-Bayoumy K: The role of selenium in cancer prevention; Can Prev 1991:1-15

70. Negri E et al: Intake of selected micronutrients and the risk of breast cancer; Int J Canc 65:140-144

71. Farrow DC: Geographic variation in the treatment of localized breast cancer;NEJM 1992;326:1097-1101

72. Bowlin SJ Leske MC Varma A et al: Breast cancer risk and alcohol consumption: results from a large case-control study; Int J Epidem 26:915-923, 1997

CHAPTER 5

1. Lynch HT Lynch JF: Breast cancer genetics in an oncology clinic: 328 consecutive patients; Cancer Genet Cytogenet 23:3690-72 1986.

2. Laing AE Demenais FM Williams R et al: Breast cancer risk factors in african-american women: The howard university tumor registry experience; The J Natl Med Assoc 1993;85:931-39.

3. Marcus JN Watson P Page DL et al: The pathology and heredity of breast cancer in younger women; NCI Monographs. 1993)

4. David KL Steiner-Grossman P: The Potential use of Tumor Registry data in the recognition and prevention of hereditary and familial cancer; NY State J Med 91:150-152, 1991.

5. Claus EB Risch N Thompson WD: Autosomal dominant inheritance of early onset breast cancer; Cancer 73:643-51 1994.

6. Gail MH Brinton LA Byar DP et al: Projecting individualized probabilities of developing breast cancer for white females who are being examined annually; J Natl Cancer 81:1879-85 1989.

7. Vogel VG Batiste RG: Increasing the Use of Screening Mammography Among African American Women; Breast Dis. A Yr Book Quart. 3:4 1992

10-11.

8. Hoskins KF Stopfer JE Calzone KA et al: Assessment and counseling for women with family history of breast cancer: A guide for clinicians; JAMA 273:7 577-85 Feb 15 1995.

9. Shiao YH Chen VW Scheer WD et al: Racial disparity in the association of p53 gene alterations with breast cancer survival; Can Res 55:7 Apr 1 1485-90 1995.

10. Muss HB Thor AD Berry DA et al: c-erbB-2 expression and response to adjuvant therapy in women with node-positive early breast cancer; NEJM 330:1260-1266 1994.

11. Freeman HP Wasfie TJ: Cancer of the breast in poor black women; Cancer 1989;63:2562-2569.

12. Visco F: It is wrong to test women outside research protocols; Medical Tribue September 5, 1996 p 10.

13. Spiegelman D Colditz GA Hunter D Herzmark E: Validation of the gail et al model for predicting individual breast cancer risk;JNCI 86(8) April 20, 1994

14. Weiss HA Brinton LA Brogan D et al: Epidemiology of in situ and invasive breast cancer inwomen aged under 45; Br   Cancer 73:1298-1305 1996

CHAPTER 6

1. Holleb AI Venet L Day E: Breast cancer detected by routine physical examination. NY State H Med 60:823-827 1960

2. Shapiro S Strax P Venet L: Periodic breast cancer screening. Arch Environ. Health 15:547-553, 1967

3. Strax P: The Guttman Institute story. In: Strax P ed Control of Breast Cancer Through Mass Screening. Littleton, Massachusetts PSG Publishing Co., 1979; 183-187

4. Shapiro S Venet L Strax P: Prospects for eliminating racial difference in breast cancer survival rates;A J Pub H 72:10 1142-1145 Oct 1982

5. Breslow L:Final reports of national cancer institute ad hoc working group on mammography screening for breast cancer and a summary report of their joint findings and recommendations. Epidemiology-biostatistics working group. DHEW Publication No. (NIH) 77-1400 Washington D C: Govt Print Office, 1977

6. Strax P, Venet L, Shapiro S:Mass screening in mammary cancer;A J Pub H 23:875-878 April 1969

7. National Cancer Institute SEER Program 1973-1981

8. Black americans' attitudes toward cancer and cancer tests: Highlights of a study. Ca-Cancer J for Clinicians 31:4 July/Aug 1981

9. Dodd GR Fink DJ Murphy GP: Breast cancer detection and community practice;Executive summary report of a workshop cosponsored by the general motors cancer research foundation and the american cancer society. Ca-Cancer J for Clinicians 39:4 July/Aug 1989

10. Remington PL Lantz PM: Using a population-based cancer reporting system to evaluate a breast cancer detection and awareness program. Ca-Cancer J for Clinicians 42:6 November/December 1992

11. Kaufmam AJ Worrell J Bain RS et al: American cancer society's breast cancer detection awareness program: the 1988 middle tennessee experience. Sout Med J 83:618-620,1990

12. Lynch HT Fitzgibbons Lynch JF: Heterogeneity and Natural History of Hereditary Breast Cancer;Surg Clin of No Amer 70:4 Aug 1990 753-776

13. White E:Rising incidence of breast cancer (response to letter).JNCI 80:2, 1988

14. Fisher B Anderson S Redmond C K et al: Reanalysis and results after 12 years of followup.....;NEJM 1995;333:1456-61

15. Smart CR Byrne CB Smith RA et al: Twenty-year follow-up of the breast cancers diagnosed during the BCDDP;CA 47:3 May/June 1997 134-149

16. SEER CANCER STATISTICS REVIEW, 1973-1992 National Cancer Institute--National Institutes of Health

17. Miller AB: Mammography screening guidelines for women 40 to 49 and over 65 years old;Ann Epidemiol 4:96-101 1994

18. Chu KC Smart CR Tarone RE: Analysis of breast cancer mortality and stage distribution by age for the Health Insurance Plan clinical trial;J Nat Can Inst 1988 80:1125-1132

19. Taber L: New swedish breast cancer detection rate presented at american cancer society workshop on breast cancer detection;February 1993

20. Larson DL: Combined analysis of swedish trials presented at NCI international workshop on screening of breast cancer;Bethesda MD February 1993

21. Hendrick RE Smith RA RutledgeJH et al: Benefit of screening mammography in women ages 40-49;A meta-analysis of new randomized controlled trials results in NIH consensus development conference ...Program and abstracts Nat Can Inst 1996

22. SEER Statistics Review, 1973-1992 National Institutes of Health National Cancer Institute.

23. Janjan NA Nattinger AB Young M Wilson JF: First year treatment charges for early stage versus locally advanced breast cancer;Breast Dis 6:27-37 1993

24. Liberman L Dershaw DD Deutch BM: Screening mammography: value in women 35-39 years old;AJR Am J Roentgenol 161:53-56 1993

25. Byrne C Shairer C Wolfe J et al: Mammographic features and breast cancer risk: effects with time, age, and menopause status; J Nat Can Inst 87:1622-1629 1995

26. Mathews ED et al: Int J Radiat Oncol Biol Phys 14:659-663 1988

27. Nixon AJ Neuberg K Hayes DF et al: Relationship of patient age to pathologic features of the tumor and prognosis for patients with stage I and II breast cancer;J Clin Oncol 12:888-894 1994

28. Mettler FA Upton AC Kelsey CA et al: Benefit versus risks from mammography;Cancer 77:5 Mar 1 1996 903-909

29. Kopans DB: Mammography and radiation risk;Radiation Risk A Primer Amer Col Radiol 1996 21-22

30. Kerlikowske K Grady D Barclay J Sickles EA Ernster V: Effects of a\age,breast density, and family history onthe sensitivity of first screening mammography;JAMA 276:1 July e 1996 33-38

CHAPTER 7

1. Robinson SB Ashley M Haynes MA: Attitude of african-americans regarding prostate cancer clinical trials;J Com Health 1996 Apr;21(2):77-87

2. Weijer C Freedman B Fuks A et al: What difference does it make to be treated in a clinical trial? a pilot study;Clin Inves Med 1996 Jun;19(3):179-83

3. Gorelick PB Richardson D Judson E et al: Establishing a community network for recruitment of african-americans into a clinical trial... (editorial);JNMA 1996 Nov;88(1):701-4

4. Thomas CR Pinto HA Roach III M Vaughn CB: Participation in clinical trials: is it state-of the-art treatment for african americans and other people of color? JNMA 86(3) 177-82

CHAPTER 8

1. Fisher B Fisher ER Redmond C Brown A: Tumor nuclear grade, estrogen receptor, and progesterone receptor: their value alone or in combination as indicators of outcome following adjuvant therapy for breast can-

cer.Breast Cancer Res Treat 1986;7(3):147-60

2. von Rueden DG Wilson RE: Intraductal carcinoma of the breast. Surg Gynecol Obstet 1984 Feb;158(2):105-11

3. Fisher ER: The Pathologist's Role in the Diagnosis and Treatment of invasive breast cancer, Symposium on breast cancer, Surg Clin Nor Amer 58:4 Aug 1978 705-720

4. Beahrs OH: Staging cancer, Ca-A Can J for Physicians 41:2 March/April 1991

5. Hems G: Epidemiological characteristics of breast cancer in middle and late age. Brit J Cancer 74:226-234 1970

6. Munzarova M Kovarik J Hlavkova J Kolcova V: Course of breast cancer disease and ABO blood groups. Biomed Pharmacother 1985;39(9-10):486-9

7. Olszewski W Darzynkiewwicz A Rosen P et al: Flowcytometry of breast carcinoma: I Relation of DNA Ploidy level to histology and estrogen receptor. Cancer 48:980-984, 1981

8. Natarajan N Nemoto T Mettlin C Murphy GP: Race-related differences in breast cancer patients. Results of the 1982 national survey of breast cancer by the American College of Surgeons; Cancer 1985 Oct 1;56(7):1704-1709

9. Harris J R Morrow M Bonadonna G: Cancer of the breast. In:Devita V T Jr Hellman S Rosenberg SA. Cancer:principles and practic of oncology. 4th ed.Philadelphia:Lippincott, 1993;1264-1332

10. Lagios MD: Duct carcinoma in situ. Surg Cl of N Amer 70:4 Aug 1990 853-871

11. Weiss HA Brinton LA Brogan D Coates RJ et al: Epidemiology of in situ and invasive breast cancer in women aged under 45.BritJ Can 73:1296-1305 1996

CHAPTER 9

1. Atkins H Hayward JL Klugman DJ: Treatment of early breast cancer:a report after ten years of a clinical trial. Brit Med J 423-429 May 20 1972

2. Keynes G: Conservative treatment of cancer of the breast. Br Med J 1937; 2:643-647

3. Huggins C Dao T: Characteristics of adrenal dependent mammary cancer. Ann Surg 140:497 1954

4. Coates RJ Bransfield DD Wesley M Hankey B Eley JW Greenberg RS. Flanders D Hunter CP Edwards BK Forman M et al: Differences between black and white women with breast cancer in time from symptom recognition to medical consultation. Black/White Cancer Survival Study Group.J Natl Cancer Inst (1992 Jun 17) 84(12):938-50

5. Halstead WS: The results of operations for the cure of cancer of the breast performed at Johns Hopkins hospital from June 1889 to January 1894. Ann Surg 20:497-550 1894

6. Halstead WS: The results of radical operations for the cure of cancer of the breast. Ann Surg 46:1 1907

7. Pierquin B Baillet F Wilson JF: Radiation therapy in the management of primary breast cancer. Am J Roentgenol Rad Ther Nucl Med 127:645-648 1976

8. Crile G Jr: Simplified treatment of cancer of the breast: early results of a clinical study. Ann Surg 1961 153:745

9. Madden JL: Modified radical mastectomy: SG&O 121:6 1221-1230 Dec 1965

10. Handley RS Thackray AC: Conservative radical mastectomy (patey's operation). Ann Surg 880-882 Dec 1969

11. Meyer AC Smith SS Potter M: Carcinoma of the breast a clinical study. Arch Surg 113:364-368 April 1978

12. Fisher B: Breast cancer management:Alternatives to radical mastecto-my. N Engl J Med 301:326-329, 1979

13. Anglem TJ: Management of breast cancer:radical mastectomy. JAMA 230:1 99-105 Oct 7 1974

14. Haagensen CD: A great leap backward in the treatment of carcinoma of the breast. JAMA 224:1181-1183

15. Haagensen CD Bodian C: A personal experience with halsted's radial mastectomy. Amer Journ Surg 199:2 143-150 Feb 1984

16. Urban JA Baker HW: Radical mastectomy in continuity with enbloc resection of the internal mammary lymph-node chain. Cancer 5:5 992-1008 Sept 1952

17. Patey D: A review of 146 cases of carcinoma of the breast operated on between 1930 and 1943. Br J Cancer 21:260-269,1967

18. Delarue NC Anderson WD Starr J: Modified radical mastectomy in the individualized treatment of breast carcinoma. SG&O 79-88 July 1969

19. Fisher B Montague E Redmond C et al: Comparison of radical mas-tectomy with alternative treatments for primary breast cancer: A first report of results from a prospective randomized clinical trial, Cancer 39:2827 1977

20. Fisher B Wolmark N: Limited surgical management for primary breast cancer: a commentary on the NSABP report. World J Surg 9:5 682-691 Oct 1985

21. Crile G JR Esselstyn CV Jr Hermann RE et al: Partial mastectomy for carcinoma of the breast. SG&O 136:929-933 1973

22. Veronesi U Saccozzi R Del Vecchio M et al: Comparing radical mas-tectomy with quadrantectomy, axillary dissection and radiotherapy in patients with small cancers of the breast. NEJM 305:6-11 July 2 1981

23. Fisher B Wolmark N Fisher ER et al: Lumpectomy and axillary dis-section for breast cancer: surgical, pathological and radiation considera-tions. Wor J Surg 9:692-698 1985.

24. Fisher B Montague E Redmond C et al: Comparison of radical mastectomy with alternative treatments for primary breast cancer: A first report of results from a prospective randomized clinical trial. Cancer 39:2827 1977

25. Levene MB Harris Jr Hellman S: Treatment of carcinoma of the breast by radiation therapy. Cancer 39:6 2840-2845 June Suppl 1977

26. Rose MA Olivotto I Cady B et al: Conservative surgery and radiation therapy for early breast cancer: Long-term cosmetic results. Arch Surg 124:153-157 1989

27. Fisher B Redmond C Brown A et al: Treatment of primary breast cancer with chemotherapy and Tamoxifen. NeJM 305:1 1-11 July 2, 1981

28. Block GE Ellis RS Desombre E et al: Correlation of estrophilin content of primary mammary cancer to eventual endocrine treatment. Ann Surg 188:3 372-376 Sept 1978

29. Fisher B: A biological perspective of breast cancer: contributions of the national surgical adjuvant breast and bowel project clinical trials Ca-Can J for Physicians 41:2 March/April 1991

30. Recht A   Come SE   Henderson   IC   et al: The sequencing of chemotherapy and radiation therapy after conservative surgery for early-stage breast cancer;NEJM 334:1356-61 May 23,1996

31. Sertoli MR Bruzzi P Pronzato P et al: Randomized cooperatve study of perioperative chemotherapy in breast cancer. J Clin Oncol 1995;13:2712-21

32. Fisher B Dignam J et al: Five vs more than five years of Tamoxifen.....;J Nat Can Inst 88:1529-1542 1996

33. Vieweg J Gilboa E: Consideration for the use of cytokine-secreting tumor cell preparations for cancer treatment; Cancer Invest 1995; 13(2):193-201

34. Diehr P Yergan J Chu J et al: Treatment modality and quality differences for black and white breast-cancer patients treated in community hospitals; Med Care 27(10):942-58 Oct 1989

35. McWhorter WP Mayer WJ: Black/white differences in type of initial breast cancer treatment and implications for survival; Am J Pub Health 77(12):1515-17 Dec 1987

36. Muss HB Hunter CP Wesley M et al: Treatment plans for black and white women with stage II node-positive breast cancer;Cancer 70:10 2460-67 Nov 15 1992

37. Eley JW Hill HA Chen VW et al: Racial differences in survival from breast cancer;JAMA 272:12 947-54 Sept 28 1994

38. Fisher B Anderson S Redmond CK et al: Reanalysis and results after 12 years of follow-up in a randomized clinical trial comparing total mastectomy with lumpectomy with or without irradiation in the treatment of breast cancer;NEJM 333:22 1456-61 Nov 30 1995

39. Olivotto IA: Adjuvant systemic therapy for women with breast cancer;The Female Patient vol 21 45-52 May 1996

40. Smart CR Hartmann WH Beahrs WH: Insights into breast cancer screening of younger women;Cancer; 72:1449-56 1993

41. National Institutes of Health, National Cancer Institute, Taxol and Related Anticancer Drugs, July 1993

42. Yergan J Flood AB et al: Med Care Jul;25(7):592-603

43. Saad Z Bramwell V Duff J et al: Timing of surgery in relation to the menstrual cycle in premenopausal women with operable breast cancer. Br J Surg 1994 Feb;81(2):217-20

44. Easton DF Bishop DT Crockford GP: Genetic linkage analysis in familial breast and ovarian cancer: Results from 214 families. Am J Hum Genet 1993;52:678-701

45. Roach M Alexander M:. The prognostic significance of race and survival from breast cancer: a model for assessing the reliability of reported survival differences;JNMA 1995;87:214-219

46. Ragaz J Jackson SM et al: Can adjuvant radiotherapy..improve the overall survival of breast cancer patients in the presence of adjuvant chemotherapy..?....Proceedings of ASCO 1993;12:70. Abstract.

47. Stonelake PS Jones CE et al: Proteinase inhibitors reduce breast cancer cell invasion and proliferation;Br J Cancer;1994:69(Suppl 21):19
48. Malone W Perloff M Greenwald P Kelloff G: Progress in the development of several new chemopreventive agents...Chemoprevention Branch NCI. CCPC-93: Second International Cancer Chemo PreventionConference. APRIL 28-30 1993, Berlin, Germany. p. 47-48, 1993

49. DePalo G Veronesi U et al: Controlled clinical trials with fenetinide in breast cancer,.... J Cell Biochem Suppl 1995 22():11-7

50. Burns R McCarthy E et al: Black women receive less mammography even with similar use of primary care; An Int Med 1966;125:173-181

51. Farrow DC Hunt WC Samet JM: Geographic variation in the treatment of localized breast cancer. NEJM 1992;326:1097-101

52. Albain KS Green SR Lichter AS et al: Influence of patient characteristic, socioeconomic factors, geography, and systemic risk on the use of breast-sparing treatment in women enrolled in adjuvant breast cancer studies: An analysis of two intergroup trials. J Clin Oncol 14:3009-3017, 1996

53. Osteen RT: Selection of patients for breast conserving surgery. Cancer 74:366S-377S, 1994

54. Vernon CC Hand JW Field SB et al: Radiotherapy with or without hyperthermia in the treatment of superficial localized breast cancer: results for five randomized controlled trials. International Collaborative Hyperthermia Group. Int J Radiat Oncol Bio Phys 1996 Jul 1;35(4):731-44

55. Albertini JJ Lyman GH Cox C et al: Lymphatic mapping and sentinel node biopsy in the patient with breast cancer; JAMA 276:1818-1822: 1996

56. Giuliana AE Jones RC Brennan M et al: Sentinel Lymphadenectomy in breast cancer; J clin Oncol 15:2345-2350: 1997

CHAPTER 10

1. Tross S Herndon J 2nd Korzun A et al: Psychological symptoms and disease-free and overall survival in women with stage II breast cancer. cancer and leukemia group b; J Nat Can Inst 1996 May 15; 88(10):661-67

2. Fredette SL: Breast cancer survivors: concerns and coping;Cancer Nurs 1995 Feb;18(1):35-46

3. Waller M Batt S: Advocacy groups for breast cancer patients;Can Med Asso J 1995 Mar 15;152(6):829-33

4. Reynolds P Boyd PT Roberts S et al: The relationship between social ties and survival among black and white breast cancer patients;Can Epidem Biomarkers and Prevention vol 3 253-259 Apr/May 1994

CHAPTER 12

1. Fisher B Redmond C Brown A Wickerham DL Wolmark N Allegra J Escher G Lippman M Savlov E Wittliff J et al: Influence of tumor estrogen and progesterone receptor levels on the response to Tamoxifen and chemotherapy in primary breast cancer.J Clin Oncol 1983 Apr;1(4):227-41

2. Gylbert L Asplund O   Jurell G: Capsular contracture after breast reconstruction with silicone-gel and saline-filled implants: a 6-year follow-up [see comments] Plast Reconstr Surg 1990 Mar;85(3):373-7

3. Ersek RA: Rate and incidence of capsular contracture: a comparison of smooth and textured silicone double-lumen breast prostheses. Plast Reconstr Surg 1991 May;87(5):879-84

4. Lemperle G: Unfavorable results after breast reconstruction with silicone breast. Acta Chir Belg 1980 Mar-Apr;79(2):159-60

5. Cohen IK: Reconstruction of the nipple-areola by dermabrasion in a black patient.Plastic Reconstruction Surg 67(2) feb 1981 23-29

6. Wallace MS Wallace AM et al: Pain after breast surgery: a survey of 282 women. Pain 66:195-202, 1996

I N D E X

A

Abortion and Breast Cancer/ 65
After Surgery--Radiation or Chemotherapy/ 130
Age to Start Mammogram Screening in African American women/ 94
Alcohol and breast cancer/ 70
Anatomy of the Breast
       Blood Supply/ 19-20
       Glandular Structure/ 18
       Lymphatic Supply/ 19
       Muscles Under the Breast/ 20
Angiostatin/ 137
Antiestrogens/ 133
       Tamoxifen/ 133
       Toremifene/ 134
       ICI 182780/ 134
       Megesterol/ 134
       Raloxifene/ 134
       Vitamin A derivative, 4-HPR/ 134
Axillary Node Biopsy (Sentinel Node) /130

B

Battle for Fairness in the Care of African American Women/ 141
Battle Plan Today/ 139
Biopsy of the Breast
       Aspiration cytology (Fine needle aspiration biopsy (FNAB)/ 45
       ABBI (Advanced Breast Biopsy Instrumentation/ 48
       Core Needle Biopsy/ 45
       Mammotome/ 48
       Open biopsy/ 44
       Stereotactic Core Needle Biopsy/ 47
       Trucut needle (Baxter-Travenol)/ 46
Birth Control Pills and Breast Cancer/ 64
Body Mass Index (BMI)/ 67
Bone Marrow Transplantation/ 138
       Autologous bone marrow transplant (ABMT)/ 138
Breast Cancer Detection Demonstration Project (BCDDP)/ 89

Breast Self Examinnation (BSE)/ 28

C
Cancers associated with Breast Cancer
       Breast cancer/ 60
       Colon cancer/ 60
       Hodgkins's disease/ 60
       Ovarian/ 60
       Salivary gland/ 61
       Uterus/ 60
Cellular Patterns of Breast Cancer
       Combination Group/ 111
       Comedo Cancer/ 112
       Ductal Carcinoma in Situ (DCI)/ 111
       Infiltrating Ductal/ 110
       Inflammatory Breast Cancer/ 112
       Lobular Carcinoma in Situ/ 110
       Lobular Invasive/ 110
       Medullary, Mucinous, or Tubular/ 111
       Paget's Disease/ 112
Chemotherapy/ 119, 130-133
Clinical Trials
       Minority-Based Community Clinical Oncology Program [MBCCOP]/ 103
       Phase I Trial/ 104
       Phase II Trial/ 105
       Phase III Trial/ 105
       Phase IV Trial/ 105
       Questions to ask before joining a clinical trial/ 104
       Tuskegee Syphilis Study/ 101
Complications after treatment/ 182

D
Diagnosis of Breast Cancer
       Aspiration of a Cyst/ 44
       Blood Tests/ 48
       Bone Scan/ 48
       Chest X-ray/ 48
       Diaphanography/ 42
       Liver Scan/ 48
       Mammography/ 35, 37
           Digital Mammography/ 39

Nipple discharge/ 44
Single Photon Emission Computed Tomography
    (SPECT)/ 42
Thermography/ 40
Ultrasound/ 41
Xeroradiograph/ 38
Diagnosing Recurrence of Cancer
Breast Cancer Antigen (BCA 225)/ 49
CA 27-29 or Truquant Test/ 49
Cancer Associated Antigen (CA 15-3)/ 49
Carcino-embryonic Antigen (CEA)/ 49
Mucinoid Cancer Antigen (MCA)/ 49
Tissue Polypeptide Antigen (TPA)/ 49
Diet
and Breast Cancer/ 67
B-complex vitamins/ 69
cabbage/ 69
Calcium/ 69
copper/ 69
selenium/ 69
soybean/ 69
Vitamins C/ 69
Vitamin D/ 69
Vitamin E/ 69
zinc/ 69
Differential Diagnosis
Fibroadenoma/ 33
Fibrocystic Dysplasia/ 31
Mastodynia/ 34

E
Endostatin/ 137
Environment, Occupation and Breast Cancer/ 70

F
Fairness in Breast Cancer Care for African American Women/ 141-144
Familial breast cancer/ 79
The Claus Tables/ 80
The Gail model/ 80
Female Hormones Produced in the Body and Breast Cancer
androstenidione/ 63

estradiol/ 61
    estriol/ 61
    estrone/ 61
    prolactin/ 63

G

Genes Associated with Breast Cancer
    BRCA1/ 77
    BRCA2/ 78
    c-erbB-2/ 83
    p53/ 82
Guidelines for Breast Cancer Detection (American Cancer Society)/ 92

H

Health Insurance Plan of Greater New York (HIP)/ 85-86
    Guttman Institute and Philip Strax/ 86
Herceptin/ 137
Hormone Control of the Breast/ 21
Hormones and Chemotherapy/ 131, 133
Hormones for Hot Flashes and Breast Cancer/ 63

I

Immunotherapy/ 136
    Bacillus Calumette Guerre (BCG)/ 136

L

Lumpectomy with Radiation/ 127

M

Mammals and Breast Tissue/ 17
Marimastat/ 137
Megestrol/ 134

O

Obesity,Diet and Breast Cancer/ 67

P

Palliative treatment options/ 186
Plastic Surgery
    Silicone Implants/ 187-191

The TRAM (transverse rectus abdominis myocutaneous)
flap/ 187
Tissue Expander Technique/ 187
Pregnancy and Breast Cancer/ 66
Prognostic Indicators/ 49
DNA Index/ 51
Estrogen Receptor/ 50
Progesterone Receptor/ 50
Prostatic specific antigen (PSA)/ 51
S-Fraction/ 51

R

Racial Genetics and Breast Cancer/ 71
Duffy gene/ 72
Radiation therapy/ 127
Sequencing of chemotherapy and radiation/ 130
Raloxifene/ 134
Reach to Recovery/ 181
Rehabilitation and Complications/ 184
Risk Factors for Breast Cancer
Advancing Age/ 55
Breast Feeding/ 57
Cancers associated with breast cancer/ 60
Female Sex vs Male Sex/ 56
Fibroadenoma/ 58
Fibrocystic Dysplasia with Atypia/ 59
Heredity/ 55
Injury/ 56
Lobular Carcinoma in Situ (LCIS)/ 59
Male Sex/ 56
Obesity/ 67
Parity/ 57
Proliferative Breast Disease/ 58
Radiation/ 58
RU-486/ 136

S

Screening Projects
Breast Cancer Detection Demonstration Project
(BCDDP)/ 89
Guttman Institute/ 86
Health Insurance Plan of Greater New York (HIP)/ 85-86

Sentinel node biopsy/ 130
Smoking and Breast Cancer/ 69
Socio-economic Status and Breast Cancer/ 73
Society of Cancer Researchers Advocating Therapeutic
        Excellence for Special Populations [SOCRATES]/ 103
Staging Breast Cancer Systems
        AJCCSER (American Joint Committee for Cancer Staging
        and End Results)/ 113
        IUAC (International Union Against Cancer)/ 114
        TNM (Tumor size, Nodes, Metastasis)/ 113
Support Groups
        SisterReach Advisory Council/ 152
                LaVerne Baker/ 153
        The Arkansas Witness Project:/ 146
                Dr Deborah Erwin/ 147
        The Breast Cancer Resource Committee/ 148
                Zora Kramer Brown/ 149
        The Sisters Network/ 150
                Karen E Jackson/ 151
Surgery and the Menstrual Cycle/ 130
Surgery for Breast Cancer
        Bilateral total mastectomy/ 126
        Halstead Radical Mastectomy/ 120-123
        Lumpectomy with Radiation/ 127
        Modified Radical Mastectomy/ 123
        Partial Mastectomy/ 125

T
Tamoxifen/ 133, 157
Taxol (paclitaxel)/ 135
Taxotere/ 135
Thalidomide/ 136
The National Breast Cancer Coalition (NBCC)/ 82
Thyroid and Breast Cancer/ 66
Treatment after Surgery
        Hormones/Chemotherapy/ 131
        ICI 182780/ 134
        Megesterol/ 134
        Sequencing of chemotherapy and radiation/ 132-133
        Vitamin A derivative, 4-HPR/ 134
